HEAL   SITION

Understanding key ideas and tensions in contemporary health policy

Alan Cribb

First published in Great Britain in 2017 by

Policy Press
University of Bristol
1-9 Old Park Hill
Bristol
BS2 8BB
UK
t: +44 (0)117 954 5940
pp-info@bristol.ac.uk
www.policypress.co.uk

North America office:
Policy Press
c/o The University of Chicago Press
1427 East 60th Street
Chicago, IL 60637, USA
t: +1 773 702 7700
f: +1 773-702-9756
sales@press.uchicago.edu
www.press.uchicago.edu

British Library Cataloguing in Publication Data
A catalogue record for this book is available from the British Library

Library of Congress Cataloging-in-Publication Data
A catalog record for this book has been requested

ISBN 978-1-4473-2322-8 paperback
ISBN 978-1-4473-2321-1 hardcover
ISBN 978-1-4473-2325-9 ePub
ISBN 978-1-4473-2326-6 Mobi
ISBN 978-1-4473-2324-2 ePdf

Cover design by Hayes Design
Front cover image: istock
Printed and bound in Great Britain by Clays Ltd, St Ives plc
Policy Press uses environmentally responsible print partners

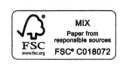

Contents

Acknowledgements   iv
Preface   v

one   Building blocks   1

two   Taking less medicine   27

three   Choosing care   55

four   Systems and lives   79

five   Especially for you   103

six   The challenge of integration   129

seven   Shaping the future   153

References   185
Index   193

Acknowledgements

Thank you to all my colleagues in the Centre for Public Policy Research for creating a warm and intellectually stimulating academic home for me. Particular thanks go to Sharon Gewirtz, John Owens, Teo Mladenov and Sara Donetto for collaborations on themes that overlap with the themes of this book. In addition John graciously agreed to read the first draft and provided me with extremely helpful comments for the revision, and Sharon and Sara helped me to finalise the manuscript.

I am also especially grateful to Vikki Entwistle, with whom I have collaborated for several years and who has read and commented on much that I have done – including this work – and has been a partner in many scholarly endeavours. At the same time that the chapters of this book were being drafted I was working with Vikki and John Owens (and others including Ian Watt, Heather Morgan, Simon Christmas and Zoe Skea) on a project focused on support for self-management. Conversations within that research team helped to sustain and motivate me – not least because of the number of treats we somehow fitted around our project meetings.

I am indebted to the Health Foundation for funding and practical support. This book project was started and finished while I have been a Professorial Fellow with the Foundation, and it is extremely unlikely that it would have been completed without that support. I would like to thank Nick Barber, Helen Crisp, the Improvement Science Fellows and the other members of the erstwhile Improvement Science Development Group. It has been a privilege to work alongside these colleagues even though I am very conscious that I have not learned as much from them as I should have done.

Of course I must, and am happy to, acknowledge my wonderful family. First and foremost thank you to Jacky for supporting me so wholeheartedly even when my work is a nuisance. But thanks also go to the entire 'Cribb and Ballard' clan, and not least to my much missed mother, Joan Ashton Cribb:

> Her gentle being was possessed by love and joy and tolerance. (Will Cribb, 2015)

Preface

Ideas are key components of health policy and health systems. They shape everything that happens and is done, including all healthcare practices. In this book I explore the ways in which key ideas about healthcare are changing, focusing in particular on the rise of a 'social', as loosely contrasted with a 'clinical', approach to healthcare. I argue that these changes – in which biomedical concerns are increasingly seen as nested within (often contentious) personal and social concerns – is part of a major historical transition. This transition is not just about the changing patterns of ill-health (with, for example, the growth in salience of long-term conditions) or even the broader social transitions manifested in trends such as the decline in deference or the rise in patient or public expectations, but is also a deeper philosophical transition in our conceptions of the nature and purpose of healthcare. While welcoming this transition I set out and explore the additional challenges that it produces for health policy, and argue that these challenges should push us towards building a 'learning healthcare system' in a very expansive sense.

In Chapter One I introduce the notion of a philosophical transition as part of a discussion about ideas being the building blocks of health policy. Using the examples of 'cure' and 'care' I illustrate the ways in which ideas are embedded in healthcare settings and practices and begin to indicate the many broader questions that surround the relationships between medicine and persons. Then, using a simplified priority-setting case, I introduce the challenges facing policy makers who, in trying to bring about 'policy futures', have to arbitrate between different visions of healthcare. Chapter Two examines the premise that health policy is 'out of kilter' and needs reform. It suggests that much of the debate about reform can be seen, in crude terms, as a debate between 'more medicine' and 'less medicine' or, more precisely, between continuing processes of medicalisation and forces of 'de-medicalisation', where the latter refers to the erosion of, or a diminished role for, a narrow focus on bodies rather than on persons. Chapter Two concludes with the discussion of a multi-dimensional account of person-centredness, seen as a contrast to a heavily biomedical model of healthcare.

Chapters Three, Four and Five focus in much more depth on themes arising from person-centred models of healthcare – patient agency, holism and personalisation, respectively. Each of these chapters highlights tensions that emerge *within* each theme – tensions between 'independent choice' and 'relational autonomy', between holism as applied to systems and as applied to persons, and between biological and biographical dimensions of personalisation. They also analyse tensions that *cut across* these themes – notably the tension between more individualist and more social conceptions of persons. The insights that animate discourses of person-centredness are invaluable – pushing us, for example, towards much broader constructions of health-related practices and actors, increasing the 'bandwidth' of conventional healthcare thinking to encompass the multiple layers – internal and external – that make people what they are; and towards understanding the potential importance of better 'tailoring' care. All these things are arguably central if we want healthcare to be effective. But at the same time these ideas, especially in combination, produce many challenges. For example, can we pursue individual autonomy and personalisation without building stronger forms of social coordination and reciprocity; and can it make sense to talk about 'person-centred' policies if these policies risk exacerbating health inequalities? In other words these chapters illustrate that person-centred models cannot be seen as simple 'solutions' to health policy problems but should, rather, be seen as a – valuable – opening up of competing policy and practice possibilities and dilemmas.

In Chapter Six I analyse the increasingly influential idea that healthcare systems, or health and social care systems more broadly, need to be better integrated – that both services and the experiences of individuals need to be less 'fractured' and that this depends upon attending to the overall architecture of systems. While strongly endorsing this idea I unpack different conceptions, elements and purposes of integration and suggest that we should go forward with a clear understanding that – because multiple value tensions pervade healthcare – such moves towards integration will inevitably involve conflict and can, for very good reasons, only ever be partial. This, I argue, is because a sufficiently rich health system must encompass currents and vantage points that are, to some degree, incompatible with one another. Nonetheless, I suggest, the aspiration towards greater integration – including the focus on system architectures and the stresses they hold together – is of critical importance.

The final chapter – Chapter Seven – asks how health policy needs to change character in the light of the transitions and tensions reviewed in the book. My suggestion is that the emphasis in health policy has to move more decisively from a delivery model to a deliberative model of healthcare; or, in other words, from an assumed model of 'top-down' service provision towards a more diffused and democratic model. I also argue that the philosophical transition that I have explored should, in part, be seen as a transition *towards* philosophy, because philosophical questions are now manifestly at the centre of healthcare debate and activity. Finally, I pull together some substantive conclusions about the key balancing acts that need to be struck in shaping the future of healthcare, including the balance between the responsibilities of policy makers and professionals, on the one hand, and the collective responsibility of patients and publics, on the other. Overall, my message is that health policy thinking is becoming more expansive and thereby more difficult and that if we care about the things we claim to – such as system effectiveness and equity – this is something we must embrace.

ONE

Building blocks

In this book I argue that healthcare is undergoing a major 'philosophical transition'. In what follows I will review this transition (beginning by outlining its nature in the next section of this chapter) and I will show why it is valuable – in brief, because it is about better connecting healthcare processes to people. At the same time I will show why this transition is extremely challenging. In summary, this is because it both brings forth and highlights fundamental dilemmas. It is commonplace for people to call for broad-ranging 'culture change' in healthcare; and I will be doing something similar. But I would argue that the 'culture change' needed is more radical than is often recognised. It means, I suggest, not only applying new sets of ideas to healthcare but also making space for very different ways of thinking.

The book explores some of the key ideas shaping, and being debated within, contemporary health policy in the relatively affluent regions of the world, sometimes simplified as the 'West' or 'Global North'. In particular I focus on ideas about the fundamental kinds of 'good things' or 'goods' at stake in health policy, the evolution of thinking about these goods and their translation into practice, and on the challenges and tensions generated by this evolution and translation. To make this agenda appear less abstract and more practical I will use the familiar ideas of 'cure' and 'care', and the contrast that is often drawn between them. We can ask: How do the ideas of 'cure' and 'care' shape health policy or practices in particular healthcare settings? What are the tensions between 'cure' and 'care', do we have the right kind of balance between them, and what further tensions are generated by trying to change the balance? Throughout this chapter I will return to these questions to introduce my main themes.

But I will begin by sketching an even more concrete and everyday example.

Like all of us Freida engages in many 'health-related practices'. She engages with health services on her own behalf and with her family and, partly prompted by her experience of supporting her sister through a long period of cancer treatment, she has even joined a local consultation group reviewing innovations in local health provision. In addition, she takes exercise and does other things to look after herself that fall outside of formal health services. This morning, for example, on the way to work, she has dropped into the pharmacist to buy some over-the-counter medicine that she knows helps her manage her sinusitis. Even before that she has rung a friend, Cory, to help her decide whether she should go into work at all. Increasing demands and targets from her employer are making her anxious and sometimes it feels as if this is unbearable and her working life is unsustainable. Talking it through with Cory always helps but they both recognise that this pattern of day-to-day coping may not be wise. A few years ago Cory took a course of prescribed drugs to help her with depression and they occasionally talk about the possibility of Freida's seeking some similar kind of medical treatment, but Cory recognises that Freida is reluctant to go down this avenue and she concentrates, in the main, on listening to Freida and on providing moral support with Freida's efforts to be OK. Today, though, Freida is feeling more optimistic – her boss is leaving and she suspects the way he treats her might exacerbate the pressures from targets and play a big part in the work-related stress. She also decides it will do her good to get out of work for 30 minutes at lunchtime and go for a run. She values the space and the exercise. Tomorrow, she thinks, she will take a 'healthy lunch' and her 'activity tracker' with her, so with these adjustments to her diet and exercise pattern, she is looking after her body too. As she walks towards her workplace she tries to form a strong resolution to take a lunch outing and not to get trapped in all day.

This description of a fragment from someone's day illustrates a few of the things that are relevant to thinking about health and health ecologies, and some of the 'goods' involved. It also illustrates some of the contrasts between different goods. Although they are both important, the help that Freida gets from the over-the-counter medicine seems very different from the help she gets from her friend. The former kind of good – a physical remedy for a physical disorder or disease – seems to operate in a way that is unmediated by human relationship. The latter kind of good – support through talking and listening – seems to operate essentially through a human relationship. The distinction between the 'medicine-taking' and the 'human support' facets of healthcare is also reflected in Freida and Cory's discussions about how Freida might best deal with her long-term anxiety. How much should she be thinking in terms of 'treatment for disease' and how much in terms of 'support for dis-ease'? In very broad terms this corresponds with the tension introduced above, and that arguably runs through all healthcare – the well-worn contrast between 'cure' and 'care'. To repeat the questions I have already raised: what difference does it make if we stress one or other of these two ideas – ideas about what healthcare is and is for – within a service or area of policy? And, assuming we think that both ideas are very important, what are the challenges of combining them?

Another issue that is thrown up by Freida's case is the question of agency – who are the actors in health policy and healthcare? How far should we think about 'health work' as the responsibility of expert or professional groups of people, or how far is it something that we all do for ourselves or for those around us? It is tempting sometimes to think of health as essentially the province of specialist workers – especially in a society with a highly developed division of labour and the extensive professionalisation of health-related roles. But both the importance of Freida and Cory's conversations and the related reflections on the workplace should remind us that this is a mistake. The Freida example says comparatively little about formal health services or health professionals, highlighting other relevant actors including Freida herself, although professionals are certainly there in the background and I will come back to them very shortly.

The Freida example also points to broader factors, sometimes referred to as the 'social determinants of health' – the things that influence her present and future health and well-being, such as her working conditions and diet and so on – and indicates that at least some of these things are not within her control. Of course a full discussion and list of social determinants would be very long and would potentially encompass everything in Freida's socioeconomic and cultural environment (including the results of her own actions). There is a sense in which if we want to 'zoom in' on Freida's health this requires us to 'zoom out' to the whole world. This provides another sense in which everyone is implicated in, and arguably shares some level of responsibility for, health policy. Policy, in this sense, is not something that simply arises from official authorities through 'top-down' processes, but is something that emerges and is shaped more diffusely. Furthermore, from this vantage point it is difficult to make clear separations between health policy and practice and other areas of policy and practice – social, economic, environmental policies and practices and so on – given that the latter have very significant implications for health.

This little case study could easily be constructed with a different emphasis that highlights official healthcare systems and health professionals. Freida may have one or more chronic illnesses (including and on top of the sinusitis) and may well have regular appointments to review and revise treatment regimes and so on, but even if she is, as yet, free from these kinds of health services routines she still has occasion to consult medical and other professional advice from time to time. Indeed all of the factors briefly reviewed here are relevant to planning health services and health-professional roles. Health services need to cater for multiple aspects of physical, mental and social well-being, and they need to be able to support and provide both 'health' and 'care'. In addition, people who plan and work in services also need to attend to broader health ecologies. This is because these broader ecologies help to shape individual and community health experiences and thereby health service agendas, and also because health services can in turn help to influence broader ecologies, including the ways in which populations live their lives.

Freida and Cory, let us imagine, discuss whether or not it is time for Freida to present her anxiety to a mental health professional and regard that as an important 'back stop' to their ongoing conversations. In addition, either or both of them might have recourse to professionally informed websites or other texts about different approaches to anxiety management. The role of professionals is relatively conspicuous in the case of the sinus medication. Lying behind, and making possible, Freida's purchase is, of course – as well as a retail system – a giant system of medical and pharmacy research and clinical practice staffed by clinical scientists, doctors and pharmacists. On other occasions Freida may have been acutely unwell and have sought clinical help and possibly had medicines or treatments that are not available without medical authorisation. Indeed all of Freida's health-related concerns may become part of the focus of formal health services – she could, for example, talk through, and sometimes may be encouraged to talk through, her life-style change plans with her doctors or other health professionals.

But starting from Freida's case and point of view allows me to underline something that has become a health-policy mantra – that there are individual persons, and groups of people, at the centre of health systems. This means that those professionals who might become involved in Freida's life will, to some degree, have to engage with, and work with, individuals such as Freida and their families, friends or care-givers. In order to be effective, professionals are likely to have to be in some sense responsive not only to the specifics of Freida's life, but also to Freida as an agent – to her agendas and preferences. The questions about agency and responsibility that I have noted are partly questions about the 'division of labour' between healthcare professionals and 'lay people' or 'patients' and so on, but they are also questions about if and how these different kinds of agents can 'work together', combine their agency and share responsibility for decisions, processes and outcomes.

I will come back to Freida later in the chapter but perhaps I have said enough already to begin to indicate how our approach to healthcare depends upon what kinds of ideas we stress. This applies not only to the 'cure versus care' question but also to the assumptions we make about what counts as health-related action and where the locus of responsibility for health sits.

The philosophical transition in healthcare

The factors briefly rehearsed through the Freida scenario evoke something important about the nature of contemporary health policy in the relatively affluent regions of the world. The health agenda has become 'open-ended' – it is not clear where it starts or finishes and lines of responsibility are also unclear. Partly this is as a result of what is sometimes called the 'health transition' or 'epidemiological transition' (Caldwell, 1993) – that is, in simple terms, the changed patterns of ill-health associated with socioeconomic development, notably a decline in the relative salience of infectious disease and a rise in the relative salience of chronic diseases (such as diabetes, cancer and cardiovascular disease), resulting in proportionately fewer acute life-threatening conditions and many more longer lives often accompanied by long-term conditions. But overlapping with this are the effects of other aspects of social change – for example, less deference to authority alongside the spread of both sceptical and consumerist dispositions, more diffusion of knowledge about health and illness, including knowledge about social determinants, which have led to changing relationships and expectations between professionals, individuals and publics. These changes in the expectations on health services are also set in the midst of broader changes in expectations about what constitutes well-being, or a good life more broadly – in particular with the normalisation of the idea that individuals should be self-determining; that is, that they should shape their own lives and environments and define what matters to them. Indeed our individual identities are themselves increasingly seen as 'self-made'. In a rapidly changing world with – at least for many people – an accelerating level of information and choice flowing from every direction, and in which traditional 'scripts' are less available (because they are seen as no longer either relevant or acceptable), then people are expected to continuously engage in 'projects of self-making' as they write and rewrite their own scripts over time (Giddens, 1991).

In this context there is a lot of talk about 'new' things needing to replace 'old' things; for example, the need for new models of professionalism and healthcare – including models that harness the participation of people and are embedded in communities. I will return to this theme in several places but, to simplify, it might be said that health policy is undergoing a slow and multi-faceted paradigm change. In other words both the epidemiological transition and the accompanying social transitions have entailed and seeded what can be seen as a more fundamental 'philosophical transition' in health policy.

This philosophical transition involves a reorientation of the relationship between the 'clinic' and the 'social world', including a shift in emphasis from the former to the latter as the locus of health-related activity. Here – roughly speaking – the 'clinic' refers to the activities associated with dedicated health settings or health professionals, and the 'social world' refers to all of the other private and public spaces in which individuals and publics pursue their lives. This reorientation produces a 'fuzzier' story about the healthcare division of labour, a social diffusion of health-related concerns, technologies and data, and the recognition of broader, more plural, conceptions of expertise and legitimacy. Partly this involves the increasing dissolution of the 'boundedness' of clinical activities and concerns, such that they can reach into every space of personal and social life. Partly it entails an extended 're-socialisation' of the clinic – with increased expectations that professionals will find themselves in dialogue with, and be receptive to, other voices and be alive to the personal and social contexts in which people experience illness, health and health services. This process involves, in essence, a renegotiation of the relationship between medicine and society.

This transition has very many policy-related and practical dimensions but it also makes sense to think of it as a 'philosophical' matter. Indeed I will be arguing in what follows that it is philosophical in two senses. First, it involves changes in the mix of ideas that shape healthcare, in particular in key ideas about the nature of healthcare – that is, what healthcare is and is for. Second, once we confront questions about whether and how new ideas can be incorporated into health systems – and how new emphases can coexist with old emphases – we discover that this involves difficult philosophical problems. In other words we discover that there are no obvious ways of answering these questions, and that empirical or technical methods are certainly insufficient for addressing them. This means, in a nutshell, that policy and practice uncertainties and dilemmas can no longer be seen as marginal complications but become part of the core business of healthcare. In other words, for everyone entangled in health policy – in whatever capacity – this transition entails new ways of seeing and new ways of thinking. That, at least, is what I will be suggesting and exploring in the rest of the book.

In the remainder of this chapter I will develop the notion that ideas are the 'building blocks' of health policy, and begin to explore the implications of recognising that key ideas in healthcare – not least our conceptions of healthcare itself – are not only in flux but also often in tension with one another. In particular – at the close of the chapter – I want to suggest that it is useful to think of healthcare planning and priority setting as less about picking from a menu of competing interventions and more about the enlargement and balancing of competing conceptions and visions of healthcare.

Health-related ideas: shaping the practices and climates of health systems

Thus far I have used the ideas of *cure* and *care* to indicate what I mean by key ideas and goods in healthcare. Although these are very general, and thus relatively vague, ideas they are also fundamentally important ones that can be used to summarise the nature and aims of healthcare – we might call them 'organising ideas' or 'foundational ideas' in healthcare. They are also strongly connected to some of the other general, but absolutely central, ideas that orient the ways we think about healthcare, such as *disease* and *well-being*, or *medicine* and *persons*. In later chapters I will discuss, and in some cases analyse, these and other such ideas, some of which have only just started to emerge in Freida's story: ideas such as *choice, participation, partnership, holism, community, responsiveness* and *personalisation*. As I have said, I am treating these kinds of ideas as the 'building blocks' of health policy and systems. This use is metaphorical only in part – the notion is that healthcare is, in very important ways, constituted by these ideas, because of the ways they can be used to frame, reframe or extend the organising principles of healthcare.

Obviously, ideas like 'cure' and 'care' do not have very simple denotations – like 'bricks' and 'mortar'. They point to general notions that can be further specified and qualified in a range of ways. But they do indicate the underlying rationale of a broad range of practices. In this sense they are more like clusters of ideas – they convey frameworks of thinking, including assumptions about underlying purposes and processes. If I am 'curing' I am trying to achieve certain kinds of ends in certain kinds of ways; that is, the broad purposes and assumptions in play will be different than if I am 'caring'. In brief, to talk of 'curing' is generally to have in mind some more or less direct physical or biological intervention into the body to counteract the effects of disease; whereas 'caring', by contrast, is a more diffuse idea that can embrace 'cure-type' responses but extends much more widely to, and emphasises, such things as physical and emotional comfort, and psychological support and responsiveness. To spell all of this out is in many ways odd, because we just 'know' this, as it were unthinkingly, when we use the language.

In this context sociologists tend to talk about 'discourses' – these are ways of talking and thinking, containing constellations of related ideas, but are also embodied in our habits, practices and social institutions. Social reality is, in this sense, made from ideas. For example – within health services and elsewhere – discourses of 'audit' and 'performance' have grown in influence. At one level these discourses can be seen as 'just' a collection of ideas – sets of linked ideas about evidence, accountability and the importance of measurability – but they have also come to shape many people's environments, practices and experiences. They are not just 'thought' but they are 'done' and 'felt' and they substantially determine what matters and what is 'real'.

The approach I am taking to health policy centres on these kinds of building blocks – organising ideas and the discourses that surround them – and asks how policy is shaped by them and how they can and might be combined together. The underlying notion is that the new directions health systems are taking reflect the ways we interpret, combine and apply key ideas about health-related goods, and that these goods are not always and everywhere compatible with one another but can generate tensions that need to be acknowledged and addressed.

Of course health systems are not wholly built out of ideas. There is also the question of how ideas are practically and materially realised. We can explore this by sticking, for now, with the contrast between 'cure' and 'care'. If we talk, in broad terms, about 'curing environments' and 'caring environments' (leaving aside for a moment the issue of how far these can and should be thought about separately), then such environments are created from multiple kinds of things. These include physical structures and objects, specialist and general equipment, guidance, information and protocols on forms and software, working schedules and templates, staff and patient norms and relationships, professional routines, individual habits, attitudes and activity. Ideas – like 'curing' and/or 'caring' – can be embodied in and reproduced by all of these things.

We can imagine environments that correspond fairly closely to archetypes of cure and care (such as an acute medical unit and a long-term nursing home). These would be made up of rather different versions of the same kinds of things: the physical 'stuff', the protocols and the individual routines would reflect and realise the underlying purposes (or emphases) of the units. Of course these archetypes are crude. It will often be better not to talk of 'cure' but of 'treatment' aimed not to eliminate disease but to reduce its length, severity and impact. Furthermore, in practice there is no tidy distinction between cure and care – they need not occur in separate spaces or stages. This separation can be implied in the way, for example, that the move from 'unsuccessful' cancer treatment to 'palliative care' is sometimes spoken about. But, of course, the boundaries here are both unclear and variable. Palliative care can be combined with treatments and, indeed, forms of clinical treatment are used for palliative purposes. Nonetheless, there are sometimes well-recognised problems in this area when it comes to combining cure and care together – either in achieving the best mix of the two or in smoothly shifting the emphasis between the two. For example, there can be an unwarranted reluctance on the part of some professionals to accept the failure of curative therapy. There can also be cases of poor coordination between professionals or services with different emphases, or even just poor understanding by some of what is demanded by palliative care, including inadequate insight into the situation or experience of the person being treated (Kaur and Mohanti, 2011).

Thus these very broad-brush ideas of cure and care can be used, albeit somewhat crudely, to indicate some of the possible divergences between 'healthcare worlds'. The recognition that these different ideas will tend to produce different environments and norms is useful: (a) for showing how ideas, and the goods they represent, are central to the production of health systems; (b) for showing that different ideas cannot always, or easily, be seamlessly combined together. Ideas like cure and care – and the other ones we will be considering – need to be translated into real-world environments and actions, and generally speaking environments and actions will tend to embody some ideas (and related approaches and purposes) better than others.

I do not see this focus on ideas or discourses as a replacement for the various other ways in which health policy can be analysed, nor as sufficient unto itself – it needs to be consolidated with other approaches. Policy analysis typically considers health systems and their architectures – for example, the composition, configuration and structure of services, or of forms of funding. My emphasis is more on the architecture of our thinking about healthcare. This is another way of talking about what I earlier called the 'rationale' or 'frameworks of assumptions' conveyed by ideas. The point is to underline the way in which frameworks of thought and assumptions shape and structure activities just as design blueprints shape and structure the artefacts that are built by reference to them; or – to use an even more materialist comparison – in ways that are analogous to the shaping and structuring of biological organisms by underlying genetic codes. Authors use a number of terms to draw attention to underlying frameworks or rationales. I will draw on two of these most frequently: 'models' (for example, in relation to biomedical models or person-centred models of healthcare), and the language of 'logics' (for example, the logic of professionalism, the logic of choice, and service logic, all of which will be discussed in the following chapters).

The architectures of health ideas and of health services are overlapping determinants of practice. For example, some health policy work centres on the ideological contests between different modes of funding and organising healthcare. Other work looks at the challenges of identifying and delivering both efficient and equitable approaches to healthcare resource allocation. These currents of work on the properties and priorities of 'real world' systems are very important and I will not be ignoring them completely, but just de-emphasising them, in what follows.

I am suggesting that one approach to understanding health systems and services is to pay attention to 'organising ideas' – the underlying mix of ideas about the nature of healthcare that help to shape and structure them – and to ask how these ideas are, and should be, evolving. A particular health service unit might, for example, have to undergo a transition so as to better incorporate palliative care within and alongside its curative work. In the book as a whole I am arguing that health systems are undergoing an analogous, but more fundamental and wholesale, philosophical transition. When I come back to discussing this transition in later chapters I will largely drop the language of 'cure' and 'care'. This distinction is only one very approximate indication of another very broad-brush distinction that I have already mentioned and will consider at much greater length – the distinction between the clinical and the social dimensions of health and, more specifically, between 'biomedical' and more 'person-centred' models of healthcare.

Trends, reforms and 'trade-offs'

Social commentators make reference to broad policy trends, and these can be presented as more or less inexorable. In relation to health policy, for example, these would include, in addition to the struggle over the rising costs of care, the ever-expanding role of technology. A full account of major trends in 'developed' health economies would take a lot of space but it would include some of the things already alluded to – demographic change, including an ageing society and the growing numbers of people living with long-term conditions and multiple conditions (compared with the relative decline in the routine threat of infectious diseases); higher public expectations, including expectations of steady scientific and technological advances; and increasing demands for, and access to, both knowledge and participation or 'involvement' in various senses. This is a world in which the nature of healthcare, including the relationship between medicine and other aspects of social systems, is evolving. I will not attempt to review all such trends in this book but I will be discussing some of them in more depth in subsequent chapters. We need to recognise and understand these trends if we are to make sensible policy.

Thinking about health policy thus involves developing a sense of the broad landscape, and the direction of travel, of healthcare and broader health ecologies. But it must also include attending to the various ways in which actors can, and are positively trying to, shape this landscape and direction of travel by attempts to 're-form' health systems. Some of these reform attempts will positively celebrate, and attempt to build upon, broad trends; others will attempt to mitigate the effects of, or even resist, trends that are seen as less desirable. Reforms may be pursued because they are seen as practically necessary or politically expedient, but typically they are pursued as, or at least presented as, technical and/or ethical improvements – such as making healthcare safer, more effective and/or more respectful, legitimate or valued by people. In other words, questions about healthcare change necessarily link to questions about the purposes and values of health systems. To ask questions about possibilities without considering the issue of desirability would be absurd. (Just as to think about desirability without an interest in what is possible is likely to be fruitless.)

Questions about what matters – about the right combination of health-related goods – are not easy ones but they are unavoidable. As we construct aspects of reforms (or trends) as more or less desirable we are taking a stand on what matters. All health-policy talk, and all health-policy analysis, connects to questions about what counts as good healthcare – including 'normative' questions about what we ought to do – even if this fact sometimes goes below the radar of consciousness. Some of the time it makes sense to suspend our interest in normative questions because there are enough other things to think about. Health policy involves descriptive, explanatory and strategic questions and, although normative questions are necessarily bound up with each of these, it is not always possible, or sensible, to try to focus on all these dimensions and questions at the same time. Some approaches to policy analysis encourage this separation. They encourage us to focus on descriptive and explanatory questions (such as what is happening and why) and use these to inform strategic questions (such as what would be the likely effects of doing x or y), whilst placing normative questions (such as which of these are more or less valuable effects) on one side. Other approaches, such as those common in critical social sciences, stress the practical and theoretical entanglement of these different kinds of questions.

Although it often makes sense to push some questions into the background, in practice it is too often the normative questions – questions about 'what matters' and what we ought to be striving for – that are treated in this way. Each emphasis has advantages and disadvantages. One of the disadvantages of pushing normative questions into the background is that we can fall into the habit of debating trends and reform policies with a fuzzy sense that we are all roughly concerned about the same things. But when we look more closely it becomes obvious that this is not right and, of course, disagreements about what we think is relatively important have substantial implications for the ways in which we understand or argue for change.

A simple – although somewhat simplistic – way of illustrating this is to think about the very extensive discussions about the respective roles of market and state organisational forms in healthcare. Debates about market versus state, or about the best combination of market and state – which form a staple of health-policy discussions – can sometimes appear to proceed as if there was only a single good at stake – 'health' or sometimes 'healthcare'. On this picture there is only one relevant kind of good to consider – a good like 'fruit' that comes in lots of shapes and sizes but is all fruit. Different interventions produce different versions of the same good in bigger or smaller quantities. This treats the matter as if it were a debate about the best ways of producing and distributing some agreed good. The good to be pursued is taken as understood but, on this reading, there are important questions to be posed and contested about the best kind of 'delivery mechanism' for that good. Anyone who has thought about health policy seriously knows that this is a misleading picture – much of what is under debate in health policy is the issue of what range of goods can and should be considered, pursued, promoted or realised through health policies. Arguments about the state versus the market in health and healthcare, if they are at all sophisticated, are arguments about the different kinds of goods that might be embedded in, produced by or inhibited by these different modes of social coordination.

It should be clear, even from the very brief discussion above of Freida's experiences, that policy actors, at whatever level they operate, need to consider a range of different kinds of 'goods'. They need to bring together, but also divide their attention between, different foci and purposes. If all of health policy could be reduced to a single overarching question – which it cannot – then the question would not be 'What is the best "delivery system" for health?' but something more like 'What patterns of social organisation and action will lead to what patterns of health and care experiences?'

However, recognising the diversity of health-system values and purposes is only the first step. Complications arise not just because there is, as it were, a very long 'list' of desirable health goods, but because policy necessarily involves having to 'choose' between items on the list. 'Choice' in this case can be interpreted as something done consciously and deliberately or as something that happens more or less unconsciously and 'accidentally'. The crux of the issue is that choices often involve 'trade-offs' of one sort or another. This issue is most often discussed within health-policy analysis under the heading of priority setting and I will shortly approach it through this relatively familiar lens. But it is worth first underlining the fact that 'trade-offs' are a general feature of all health policy and, indeed, of life itself.

There are two reasons behind the need for trade-offs. First, it arises because the various kinds of health good can be seen as *competing* – we will not have the time, or energy, or financial resource to address all of them all of the time. Sometimes doing x will mean that we will not, or may not, end up doing y – this is what economists call the 'opportunity cost' of doing x. This kind of choice is frequently discussed in economic terms, such as through the language of resource allocation, but it is, of course, a pervasive phenomenon. Each of us can live only one life and, as a result, is forced to choose to do some things and not others and to steer a 'single-track' course through all the possible lives we might lead. There are an indefinitely large number of things that a health system could do and at least some of them will be ruled out because of such practical constraints.

Second, it arises because goods can sometimes be *conflicting* – some of the things we value may not be 'combinable' (or 'compossible') with other things we value. Again, this is familiar from everyday life. I may value spending some of my summer sun-bathing but I may have been advised to stay out of direct sunshine when possible because of skin sensitivity. If we assume that I care about the health of my skin then I can be said to value both the sun and the shade. I simply cannot have everything – and this kind of tension cannot be dissolved by more resources; it would not help the situation if I had more money or a longer holiday and so on.

The same 'problem of incompatibility' applies to all of the goods that can be supported by health systems. It is not possible to provide any and every combination of things, and this would be true even if resources were completely open ended. This is a universal problem. It might be worth starting by noting its relevance to treatment decisions – that is, even the most clinically defined area of decision making. The now widely understood idea of treatments having desired effects and some non-desired 'side-effects' is a clear example. A routine element of treatment decision making is weighing up the risks and costs as well as the benefits of interventions. Doctors and patients sometimes have to decide which of two incompatible sets of risks or costs is more important.

This challenge also arises at an organisational level for people who wish to change or 'redesign' health services. To return to the cancer care example, let us suppose that someone wants to reorient a unit so that is based more on a 'care model' and less on a 'cure model'. Given the exact circumstances, this may well be a justified reform, and a very good thing overall if it is done well. But in the process – if they are to act responsibly – they will need to be aware that there is a risk of some important losses as well as gains. The same challenge arises at an even larger scale if we are seeking either to promote or to evaluate the broad philosophical transition that is reviewed in this book. When and why are new organising ideas in health policy simply to be welcomed, and when and why might we need to be cautious about welcoming them?

What should we do? Comparing futures

Freida attends the first meeting of the health consultation group she has agreed to join. It turns out to be a fascinating but also very difficult evening for her. A family have left a very large legacy to be spent on 'innovations in the promotion of health or healthcare in the local community'. A small group of trustees working with local agencies have invited proposals for projects and programmes and they have produced a short list of eight potential projects. There is a substantial sum of money but, even so, they come to the conclusion that it will not be possible to fund more than three of the proposals if the funding is to provide some element of stability for the funded work. Freida and others are presented with the details of the short-listed projects and asked to deliberate and advise – at this session and in a couple of planned follow-up meetings – on what should appear in the successful list of three. Freida leaves the meeting feeling that she has failed to contribute to the discussion in the way she would like, but also with a powerful sense that the exercise is opening up important issues.

All the short-listed projects are based on successful pilot work showing at least proof of concept and some respectable 'evidence base' (albeit using different kinds of evidence). Each has strong advocates and considerable good will behind them. In summary they are:

1   A contribution to the local 'scanner appeal', which has mushroomed in scope and now has multiple sub-streams of its own. In particular the funding of some heart scanners for a consortium of primary care doctors – who are increasingly aiming to take much routine diagnostic and monitoring work from the teaching hospital in the nearest city, but don't have all the equipment they need. The purchase of this equipment will help to support their training and provide patients with quicker reassurance or referral and less travelling time. The advocates also explain that there are costs savings to be had, over time, by the provision of non-hospital-based services – savings that will underpin other aspects of the primary care teams' work.[1]

2   The establishment of a local 'expensive drugs' fund to be able to provide a safety net in cases where the normal service has ruled out, on financial grounds, medicines that are otherwise deemed to be effective, and potentially valuable to specific individual patients, but that are not on standard formularies because of their highly contested or very poor cost-effectiveness ratio – for example, perhaps extending a patient's life for a few weeks only. Advocates cite the considerable media publicity surrounding a few controversial cases, arguing that the existence of, and flexibility enabled by, such a fund – to be used in exceptional circumstances – could, they believe, command widespread public support and be vital to the individuals concerned.

3   A large-scale local trial of smartphone telemedicine applications – which, for example, allow people to self-monitor their conditions at home, and enable doctors to extend their 'virtual' consultations, examinations and tests. Those advocating this programme describe it as absolutely central to the future of healthcare in an information age and as having countless advantages; including potential to provide personalised monitoring for patients and large-scale data collection and analysis to strengthen clinical responsiveness and planning. The trial may not show huge benefits in the short term, they accept, but it will lay the foundation for a much-improved service and will give this community a national reputation for innovation and leadership in this field.

4   A programme of recruitment and training run by and for domiciliary and hospice palliative care volunteers. The local hospice has an outstanding reputation for caring for patients and families facing the last phase of life. The volunteer-run group has increasingly collaborated with other local groups

and national charities to extend its work into people's homes but needs investment to identify and train potential volunteers. It is wary of the danger of expanding without careful recruitment and training processes – underlining the need to take new people on board carefully and extend the service with great sensitivity and proper evaluation.

5   A 'gardening for health' programme – a partnership partly sponsored by local leisure organisations and supported by a high-profile local hospital doctor and targeted at isolated people living with long-term conditions and with no access to outside space – previous experience has shown this to be an exciting area that promises physical, social and mental health benefits and community building. The scheme is heavily subsidised to make it accessible. New initiatives include an 'inter-generational' gardening project bringing school-age children and seniors together.

6   A grant to underpin the grassroots youth workers team for a few years. Local government cuts have reduced youth work to a minimum and specifically mean the imminent demise of the 'grassroots' team who work on the streets and in local spaces to spend time with, and respond to the needs of, often 'disconnected' young people – providing informal education, social opportunities and responsive support for young people's individual and collective interests, projects and struggles. The team has some powerful and passionate advocates, including former 'clients', who tell vivid stories about the difference the service makes to lives.

7   The funding of an education and training programme providing mental health and counselling education and training for local health professionals aimed at (a) building a better understanding of mental health issues and (b) building capacity for, and links with, local counselling provision. Advocates stress the relative neglect of mental health problems among the local general population and the dearth in infrastructure. This project is essentially an education one and will benefit the local community only over time, but, its advocates argue, unless the professional community is itself supported that will never happen.

8   Finally, the organisers of the meeting share a proposal to expand their ad hoc consultation exercises into a larger and more representative community health forum. The idea would be for a forum of local employers, trade unions, religious organisations and local branches of health charities to meet alongside community representatives to debate and make recommendations about health planning and provision. Their hope is to get future funding from local employers, including the health service and private sector partners, but they are looking for 24 months' pump-priming money to get the project off the ground.

Freida finds all the cases pretty convincing and can see no sensible way of differentiating between them. She is conscious of certain 'biases' – she has personally seen the benefits of the local hospice and of the grassroots youth workers and she knows from her own immediate experiences that mental health support is incredibly important; other things she knows much less about – but that just makes her feel even more wary of making a contribution to the short-listing process! As the meeting goes on things seem to get more complicated and Freida is surprised to discover that the discussion gets acrimonious at one point when people start to try to narrow the short-list – arguing that some projects should not have been included at all, and some are not worth funding or are even positively harmful; but disagreeing strongly about which projects fall into these categories. In beginning to think about the issues Freida forms a sense that what is at stake is broader and deeper than the distribution of specific financial resources, and involves understanding how broader 'resources' in general can and should be deployed for the good of health, and somehow arbitrating between different visions of healthcare and society. Freida comes away from this first meeting feeling that the decisions that she and her colleagues have been confronted with are inherently difficult ones, but also with a strong belief that the process of getting people together is the start of something important, and hopeful that the group may find a constructive way forward together.

I am not going to attempt to provide a method, and certainly not an algorithm, for addressing the challenge that Freida and the group face. The example is presented simply to illustrate some issues and complexities that I will briefly expand upon (and which, hopefully, will help us to identify with Freida's feeling of being 'stuck'). In any case, there are a number of factors that should make us hesitate to 'solve' this priority-setting exercise, some of which are specific to the example and some of which are generic.

The example opens up many lines of questioning that I will not consider here. In order to put ourselves in the shoes of those at the meeting we would, for example, probably want to know something about the family who left the legacy and what they might have had in mind, including perhaps where they got the money from (for some people that might make a big difference). More broadly, it would be important to have a much fuller notion of what the alternative sources of funding might be for the various initiatives and what the normal expectations are about funding sources and boundaries within this particular national and local health economy. In other words, we might feel that, before deliberating further, we would need the immediate and the broader context to be specified in much greater detail.

But, leaving these important contextual questions in the background for now, the group is being asked to choose between, and in some measure to bring about, different policy futures and different healthcare worlds. There are plenty of significant complications and 'balancing acts' for it to consider. The example illustrates the diversity of health-related goods and purposes. It also indicates some of difficulties of identifying what counts as a health-related good both in principle and in practice; that is, what kinds of things should health policy actors be thinking about, and how can they decide, in particular instances, whether or not specific goods will flow from interventions? Freida and her peers are being asked to make judgements about the desirability of the different options – which of them will be 'effective' in various ways, and which of them offer goods or benefits that matter the most? But they may also want to deliberate about the relative possibility of realising these goods – are the claims that their advocates make for them credible; is the knowledge needed in order to decide available? In addition, the example illustrates that different projects will benefit different groups of people and individuals, and presses home the difficulty of thinking about what is fair or equitable – which people should benefit from interventions, and whose needs or interests should come first? Here I can only briefly reflect on a few of these factors. I am, of course, using the scenario as a way of approaching the challenge of thinking about policy futures more generally. It is a very imperfect analogy, partly because it is a greatly simplified scenario, but the assumption is that policy planning entails at least the complications and 'balancing acts' mentioned here.

It is worth highlighting the diversity of the goods under consideration. All of the proposed 'innovations' connect with the philosophical transition discussed above. That is, they can be seen as being about better ways of joining the 'social world' to the 'clinical world'; but they contribute to the 'join' in different ways. Some of them might be seen as about a stronger community locus for clinical agendas (such as supporting community-based equipment, local monitoring of people's daily functioning); others are more about displacing immediate clinical agendas by broadening and complementing them with longer-term health and well-being agendas (such as youth work and gardening initiatives). This difference may well be what gives rise to heated disagreement in the meeting. It is easy to see how some people could be dismissive of the longer-term projects as 'nice but not necessary' – these 'non-medical' initiatives, some might argue, should not even be in the frame because they do not qualify properly as healthcare. But other people might wish to prioritise these precisely as embodying a necessary change of perspective and emphasis. Healthcare, they might argue, should not be defined around medicine or professional roles and agendas but should involve many community members and support people to live their lives in ways that are good for them – both because this contributes to prevention or long-term health and also because it is ultimately what makes health worth pursuing. The way the priority scenario is constructed means that the projects and related goods are, by definition, 'competing'; but the possibility of strong disagreement among well-intentioned people indicates that they may also be in some deeper sense 'conflicting', that is, that they might be viewed, at base, as embodying different visions of healthcare systems. The values that are built into the different proposals mean that it is conceivable that even the availability of very many more resources, such that all of the initiatives could be funded, would not put an end to some of the disagreements.

There are various tensions underlying this priority-setting scenario. First is the tension discussed above between 'cure' (or treatment) and 'care' as two key facets of healthcare. Second are the related contests between the multiple versions of 'health' in play in the different proposals – some relating specifically to 'disease management' and others to much broader ideas such as emotional or social well-being, including the promotion of 'public mental health' in a proactive way and not just the management of mental health problems when they arise (MIND, 2016). Third is the more general problem of shorter-term versus longer-term thinking: some of the initiatives appear to be immediately directed to addressing the current needs of the local population, whereas others have a more distant and mediated relationship to that purpose, for example they are to support not only prevention but also education, research or public participation. Fourth, some of the kinds of goods under consideration seem to be relatively 'pre-defined' and fixed whereas others seem to be relatively responsive and open ended (compare the provision of expensive drugs with the open-ended conception of youth work). Finally, and linked to all of the other four, some of the goods seem to fit the idea of 'outcomes' or 'products' – brought about by health system inputs – and others seem to be more about valuable 'processes' – where the goods are intrinsic to, and embedded in, the practices themselves.

For some people it will be tempting to imagine that there might be a common denominator by which we could compare the value of each of these kinds of good and thereby the potential contribution of each of the proposed projects. On that logic we could then, perhaps, simply pick the three that scored the highest in terms of their 'productivity'.

Something like this approach is often adopted in health economics when different interventions are compared for the 'quality-adjusted life years' (or QALYs) they generate. But although this approach has some credibility and plausibility within a clinical priority-setting exercise – at least when we are comparing similar kinds of interventions for the same or similar ends – it seems very much less relevant and credible when the kinds of good at stake are so diverse. There is no reason to suppose that there is any common denominator through which the various kinds of 'outcomes' and 'processes' could be compared. This is most obvious in the case of the community health forum: the idea of the forum is to make sure that there is an element of 'ownership' of, and participation in, local health policies. This would mean that policy directions might be more representative of the population that the policies are meant to serve and might be informed by a degree of democratic deliberation. The value of 'democracy', or of 'participation' more broadly, is on a different axis from the value of the 'health outputs' themselves, such that to suggest that the sole measure of the success of participation should be whether it results in more 'health output' is to misunderstand its nature. Indeed the projects considered as a whole seem to consist of very different kinds of activities and practices, with very different kinds of underlying rationales. Considering them collectively appears to be much less like comparing alternative treatment modalities for the same condition and much more like comparing needlepoint, opera and cricket.

Even without resorting to the idea of a common denominator, in a technical or mathematical sense, there is something very tempting, and in practice something very persistent, about the notion of 'reducing' the range of health policy ends to one end, 'health'. The idea of health is so porous, and can apparently be indefinitely expanded. This is not only because we can use it to refer to both narrow conceptions of health (typically biomedically defined, and roughly equated to 'absence of disease') and broad notions of health (including various versions of positive 'well-being') but also because even if we confine ourselves to a narrow conception of health such a lot of other factors cluster closely around it because they are either (or both) causes or consequences of health. This makes the task of drawing the boundaries of healthcare (or even more broadly the health system) particularly difficult and slippery. It is far from clear what should and should not be included. For example, let us imagine – something that is plausible – that some people at the meeting question whether the activities of grassroots youth workers contribute to health, then advocates for their service might talk in terms of its contribution to the personal well-being of the young people. But if that does not seem sufficiently convincing to sceptics, then advocates could also talk about the ways in which the lives and circumstances of their clients would otherwise put them at risk of increased morbidity in the longer term, or might even point to instances of supporting them to access specific clinical services which contribute directly and immediately to their physical or mental health (and thereby also to their broader well-being). This elasticity and slipperiness, and also the 'tactical' question about how service advocates should best describe the way services promote health or well-being are pervasive features of health-policy debates.

The point I am hoping to illustrate is that we cannot make progress with debates about policy futures – even in a highly simplified scenario – without confronting the question of what healthcare is and is for. That is, without entering into debates about what I have called the 'organising ideas' that shape healthcare, or the underlying frameworks of thinking that inform healthcare policies and practices. Most simply, and most centrally, what do we think counts as 'health' and what counts as 'care'? In the consultation group scenario this need for questioning and debate about these foundational matters applies both to the advocates of different projects and to the group members. What conceptions of healthcare are the advocates really advancing, and what conceptions do group members have in mind when they are trying to make comparisons and judgements?

In the next chapter I will develop my account of the broad transition that is arguably taking place as models of 'person-centred care' increasingly compete with 'biomedical models' as organising ideas for healthcare. This transition, and the tensions it entails, provides the central theme of the book. However, there are other very important debates about the right bases for policy directions, including about the right values and visions for healthcare, that I will say less about but which overlap with my central focus on conceptions of healthcare. The conflicts in the consultation exercise illustrate that a different conception of healthcare is necessarily bound up with different notions of what counts as 'success' – including, for example, what counts as relevant evidence, effectiveness and equity.

Each of the proposers is imagining possible futures and suggesting steps to bring such futures about. But why should anyone take them seriously? Advocates will cite different amounts and kinds of evidence to support their future-oriented claims. Some activities will have been studied and evaluated more fully and systematically than others, and judgements will be made about the 'quality' of different kinds of evaluations and the corresponding 'strength' of the evidence base. This might provide one means of differentiating between the claims of the different initiatives. Up to a point this makes sense – we can and should be more sceptical about some claims than about others and there are relevant conceptions of rigour that we can bring to bear in making these discriminations. However, this is far from a straightforward business. Different kinds of research are relevant to evaluating different claims and these have correspondingly different conceptions of evidence and rigour. There are well-established and accepted approaches to measuring reductions in mortality and morbidity, and the risks of clinical side-effects, and there are often relatively clear causal lines to be drawn between clinical interventions and such positive and negative effects. The result, at least in those cases where there are large numbers of people being treated in the same way, is the ability to make some robust claims about clinical effectiveness. In other areas – such as 'emotional well-being' or 'community building' – it is more difficult to know how we would go about assessing something. Both the good in question and the causal story are much more blurred, there is often little scope for generalisation and, by no means least, all of the problems of studying open-ended, complex and shifting social systems come into play.

These differences give rise to a commonplace problem: how can we apply the same frame of reference to, let alone compare and weigh together, a case for something which is supported by clear measurements and a case for something else which is lacking such firm measures but which is instead based on other kinds of evidence, perhaps a plausible qualitative narrative? There is a danger of being misled by a plausible narrative – it may turn out to disguise a lot of things that matter. There is also an increasingly well-recognised danger in prioritising something just because it can be or has been measured. To take an example from everyday life, it would surely be straightforwardly stupid to select a friend or partner based on measurable factors such as height or size of bank balance because we didn't know how to measure factors such as kindness or integrity. (And this also suggests that there may be something problematic about calls to make everything equally measurable – would we really be better off spending time devising and applying measurements of kindness?)

However, even if we could compare all health-related action in terms of measurable 'outputs' it would not follow that we should focus on optimising the 'productivity' of such actions, that is, the 'overall output' (however construed) of the system. This would be to ignore a set of concerns that many would see as central to debates about priority setting – concerns about equity or fairness. This is a highly contested area with various different conceptions of equity available and a great deal of correspondingly complex ideological debate. I will illustrate just one aspect of this debate very briefly here. For example, if we start from an idea such as 'need' or 'disadvantage', there does not seem to be any single (shared) sense of what these things might mean.

Let us imagine that some of the acrimony at the meeting began because someone suggested that the funding should go to those with the greatest needs and interpreted this as the people who would benefit from the proposed expensive drugs fund by having their lives extended a little. But others disagree with this assessment – some saying that this life extension is valuable but not as valuable as broader and longer-term benefits for many more people, and some arguing that such life extension is sometimes wrong and 'uncaring' and that even the terminally ill as a group could have the money spent on them much more wisely by better funding of the palliative care volunteer service. Another view might be that the beneficiaries of the youth-work service and some of the older people who are attending the gardening for health programme are actually the most in need – because they are in many cases the most impoverished, facing multiple economic and social hardships, often including feelings of being disconnected from and unvalued by those around them, and with very little alternative provision made for them. Those who take this line might argue that other potential beneficiaries are relatively privileged and have many other options for promoting their physical and mental well-being. Each of the parties in these kinds of disputes seem to have a good *prima facie* case for being taken seriously. This is because there is a range of plausible but competing theories about what equity or social justice is and entails – what facets of social life and kinds of goods it should focus on, what it demands (for example, equalising distributions, guaranteeing minimum levels, rectifying historical inequalities and so on) and how it should be weighted against other concerns.

Although priority setting is important in its own right, and relevant to my focus, I am not directly concerned here with these dilemmas in the context of priority setting. The example and the brief analysis I have offered, albeit in a simple way, just serves to introduce and capture a fraction of the complex landscape and balancing acts that health-policy actors face. But it is worth noting that those who do focus on priority-setting questions draw on two broad kinds of approaches (often in combination) to addressing them that have broader relevance for health policy making. One approach is to develop measures and to refine algorithms (such as QALYS) to better enable us to use quantitative indicators to inform policy judgements, and to make comparisons, where this is meaningful and practicable, between disparate kinds of interventions and activities. There is a limit to how far this first approach can take us, both because not everything is equally amenable to measurement and because measurement cannot solve (although it can disguise) the inherent value contests in assessing and comparing different kinds of goods. A contrasting approach is to think about how priority-setting deliberations might be conducted in ways that are procedurally defensible; that is, by ensuring that the range of different legitimate perspectives is aired, heard and considered fairly. This means consideration being given to the conditions under and processes by which decisions are made as, most notably, advocated under the 'accountability for reasonableness approach' (Daniels, 2000): that is, is the process of deliberation open to public view? Are the reasons that are advanced and that shape decision making relevant? And are decisions open to revision in the light of new evidence and arguments? Both of these approaches have something to offer. I will not be looking further at the uses of devices such as QALYS in this book but I will return to the value of dialogue and deliberation, in contexts where technical measurement meets its limits, in the final chapter. For now I hope that I have underlined not only the immense difficulty of these judgements but the need to look beyond, and behind, the selection of individual projects and programmes.

In the end, the prioritisation of competing programmes of activities depends upon a thorough engagement with context (which we had provisionally set aside), including an analysis of the overall health system and ecology – what combinations of goods do and should this support? It also involves the 'prioritisation' of competing visions of healthcare and the broader health system. To recognise that there is not always a 'common denominator' by which we can objectively compare a range of different kinds of interventions – because potential interventions reflect very different conceptions of health-related action and underlying assumptions about purposes and processes – is itself an important step forward. In this respect Freida's feelings of uncertainty are a necessary step in a process of enlightenment. I will return to this notion towards the end of the book (in Chapters Six and Seven).

Conclusion

One way of summing up the ground I have covered in this chapter, and will develop further in what follows, is to start from the Institute of Medicine's framework on quality, which states that good healthcare is 'safe, effective, patient-centred, timely, efficient and equitable'. If we want to assess whether what we offer is effective and efficient – and this seems to be of central importance – then we need to wrestle with claims and disputes about diverse 'outputs' and related evidence. There are, as just indicated, also very important disputes about the nature of equity that are again partly about evidence but also partly about the different possible interpretations of the term. Similar challenges apply in relation to some of the other terms (I will be saying more about the idea of patient-centredness in the next chapter). But there is another more fundamental sense in which this version of good-quality healthcare is open to interpretation, namely this: If I say good quality X is safe and effective, then I have not said anything at all about what 'X' is. Arguably, good-quality education, building or ballroom dancing will also be safe and effective. This account of good-quality healthcare tells us very little indeed unless we combine it with a relatively clear picture or vision of what 'X' is. It is this idea of what healthcare is and is for – in short, our conception of healthcare – that, I am suggesting, is undergoing a philosophical transition. Questions about effectiveness, equity and so on and questions about the nature of healthcare all matter, but it is disagreements about the last of these that are most easily overlooked.

Making decisions about the spread and balance of future policies and activities forces questions on us about the kind of society we want to live in and the kinds of society that we think are possible. This is more than, and different from, 'weighing up' the relative contribution of individual services. It requires us to ask some exceptionally difficult questions about the future and the combinations of goods that are possible and desirable. Furthermore, these are not just difficult empirical questions (questions for the social sciences in their descriptive, explanatory or predictive modes) but they are also inherently normative questions of ethics and politics. Only a foolish person would rush to specify and answer these questions. But we do need to make an attempt to ask the right questions and to work our way towards answering them. In this book I am hoping to make a contribution to the formulation of the relevant questions: first, by helping to highlight the broad philosophical transition we are in the midst of negotiating; and second, by seeking to uncover and illuminate some of the contests that are built into the transition – most specifically the normative tensions that need to be acknowledged and addressed as the relationships between the clinic and the wider social world are redrawn.

The Preface contains an overview of the structure of the book, but, in summary, it can be seen as having three broad 'parts'. This chapter and the following one introduce the context and nature of what I have called the philosophical transition, including (in the next chapter) the rise and significance of 'person-centred' models of healthcare. In Chapters Three, Four and Five I focus in more closely on the promise of, and potential problems produced by, person-centred models. To close the book, in Chapters Six and Seven I look to the future, asking, in particular, about the challenge of system integration and the difficulty of mobilising and 'holding together' different actors, perspectives and models. To conclude, I suggest that the transition under review requires us to build a 'learning healthcare system' – where this term is construed in a very expansive sense.

Note

[1] For example, see www.scannappeal.org.uk/, including the 'heartworks' heart scanner training tool.

TWO

Taking less medicine

It is often argued that the direction of health policy needs to change. This is only to be expected as times and circumstances change and as our understanding of things evolves. In the affluent health economies that I am focusing on here this is typically expressed in relation to changing population and disease patterns. The UK National Health Service (NHS), for example, is frequently criticised as no longer being suited for a changed world. Richard Smith, a former editor of the *BMJ*, has expressed this in blunt and forceful terms: 'When the NHS began in 1948 it made lots of sense. People suffered from infectious diseases that could be diagnosed, treated, and cured. Spending on the NHS meant that some people who would have died or been severely disabled could be returned to full health. There's not much of that now. This is the age of chronic disease, where doctors are patching up not curing, and some people (even, I suggest, many) are kept alive when it might be better for everybody, including themselves, if they were dead' (Smith, 2015).

Smith – as someone who has spent time close to the heart of medical thinking – is here aligned with those sceptics who are wary of the presumption that an increased level of clinical intervention is necessarily a good thing. On this account it seems that a service designed for wholly good purposes and staffed by conscientious professionals may nonetheless end up doing things that are, in effect, 'uncaring', and may not be providing people with either what they want or what might be seen as in their best interests. In essence, what lies behind the more or less continuous calls for 'person-centred' reforms is this recognition – that services do not always provide what we think does or should matter to people.

Here I am just using the expression 'person-centred' in a very loose way to signal the various respects in which health policies and services might better reflect, benefit and 'suit' the people they are intended to serve. (At the end of the chapter I will begin to unpack the idea of person-centredness more fully.) As noted in the last chapter, demands for reform reflect broader social changes, including in public expectations and values, as well as in disease patterns. For example, the decline in social deference and the routine questioning of most forms of social authority, including professional authority – along with broader socioeconomic changes such as the ascendancy of consumerist norms – have made unqualified medical paternalism unviable, or at least conspicuously problematic. Another important development is the increased understanding of the persistence, and in some cases the intensification, of health inequalities despite increasingly extensive healthcare provision. It has become public knowledge, and not just specialist epidemiological insight, that people's very different health experiences and opportunities are a product of broader and longer-term social determinants and that these underlying health inequalities simply cannot be satisfactorily addressed by clinical services alone. Each of these things, and many other accompanying changes, demands new directions or emphases for policy.

The book as a whole is organised around the notion that health policy involves managing the push and pull of conflicting visions of healthcare, associated health goods and models of care – for example, as in the above critique of the NHS, the potential tensions between 'treatment' and 'caring'. Sometimes these normative tensions come to the surface and are manifest in policy debates, but very often they remain below the surface. Nonetheless the forces that operate below the surface – because they operate at the foundational level that shapes and structures healthcare – have very substantial implications for the different directions in which policy and practice evolve.

In this chapter I will more fully introduce and illustrate the kinds of tensions I have in mind. To do so I will use the simplifying device of postulating one very general normative tension – which can be seen as running through many others – namely, the tension between 'medicalisation' and what might be called 'de-medicalisation'. Crudely, how far are the problems of health policy best addressed by more medicine or by less? I should stress that this is by no means a clear or a single question – it relies on a very fuzzy and, in some respects, an artificial distinction. But, allowing for its over-simplicity, this question can help to provide a broad framework for approaching foundational struggles in health policy. As will become clear, 'medicalisation' here does not refer to a simple or single thing but encompasses various strands and dimensions. And I am using the idea of 'de-medicalisation' in the same spirit – to pick out a cluster of processes and possibilities. Indeed there are not just tensions between these two very general tendencies in health policy, but equally important tensions within these tendencies.

In what follows I will further explore the suggestion that healthcare has been on the wrong track and needs redirecting and I will introduce some of the kinds of reorientation that have been advocated or are underway. First I will begin to unpack the elements of medicalisation and then I will go on to indicate how these are connected to the idea that health policy is 'out of kilter'. At the end of the chapter I will indicate how the broad aspiration towards 'person-centred care' – which can be used as a shorthand to signal an alternative to medically dominated thinking – is itself internally complex and, rather than providing simple 'answers', points in a number of different directions and raises further complications (that are followed up in the subsequent chapters). The tone of much of this chapter, with its focus on 'the wrong track', may thus appear quite negative, but it does not need to be read in that way. Each and every criticism of a conception of healthcare is, at the same time, a clue towards an alternative conception. In saying that an approach to healthcare falls short because it does not embody (a) and (b) we are implicitly arguing for a version of healthcare that does embody (a) and (b).

What's wrong with medicine?

Those who, in various respects, advocate what I am referring to as 'de-medicalisation' are not calling for the abolition of the medical profession, or even for fewer doctors. Indeed it is very often doctors themselves who make the call that I have in mind. In essence, what is being asked for is a reduction in the relative influence of a historically important current within medicine – often called 'the biomedical model'. The problem that is being highlighted – assuming that we accept it as a problem – is the danger of making sense of, and responding to, health and well-being agendas too much in terms of what is usually described as a 'narrow' or 'reductionist' approach to health. This narrow model has various facets, each of which can be characterised in various ways, but I will briefly indicate four facets. First, there is a tendency for those influenced by the biomedical model to focus on the body, or more broadly on the physical basis of health (including the physical basis of mental health) rather than on 'persons' in some general sense that encompasses the psychological and social dimensions of health. Second, there is a tendency for 'medicine', in this narrow sense, to be primarily oriented towards 'disease management' – especially cure of, or treatment for, diseases – rather than towards broader purposes such as 'health promotion' or the care and support of people. Third, there is a tendency for a 'scientistic' and instrumental, problem-solving, mindset to dominate thinking – and for problem solving to be defined in terms of finding the right technical (and often technological) intervention. Fourth, there is a tendency to assume that the professional knowledge and social authority of clinicians should be centre stage, rather than for broader conceptions and kinds of expertise and social authority to be stressed. These four facets generally cohere together because the focus on managing the 'diseased body' – the first two facets – underpins the stress on clinical intervention and authority – the second two facets.

The combined effects of these features is both powerful and pervasive in health arenas. On an individual basis we are arguably sometimes too ready to see our own concerns and experiences of ill-health through biomedical lenses. For example, when we seek a drug prescription for an ailment when something else – some form of life-style adjustment, a course of exercise or counselling, or perhaps just a reframing of the experience or change of attitude – might be better for us. On a general, global or systems basis we might come to analogous conclusions – being concerned that too many of our health-related institutions, social norms, practices and ways of thinking are framed by biomedical assumptions. For example – to echo comments that have been made by many – we may worry that we have a 'disease service' rather than a 'health service'. This, at least, is what some of the advocates of 'less medicine', in the way I am using it here, would suggest.

Even from this short sketch it should be clear why the biomedical model is often described as reductionist. The idea is that it leaves out or plays down a lot of factors and considerations that are relevant to health and well-being – for example, some 'broader' aspects of persons and social life and multiple forms of expertise – and places heavy emphases on other sets of considerations – for example, diseases and physical treatments. Calls for de-medicalisation are calls to weaken, undo or reverse these reductionist tendencies. They are asking for a reshaping of health policy around different kinds of entities, actors and actions and different forms of knowledge (that is, asking for what philosophers refer to as ontological and epistemological shifts in healthcare).

Many of the most important reforming currents in contemporary health policy might be viewed as de-medicalising ones. They include: (i) health-promotion policies and actions aimed at producing physical environments and social climates to prevent disease, enable healthier life-styles or positively promote well-being; (ii) an increasing emphasis on cross-sectoral and inter-professional working (ensuring that healthcare draws on the expertise not only of doctors, nurses and other 'allied professions' but also of those coming from outside the biomedical model, such as architects or social workers); and (iii) persistent pleas for 'partnership working' with patients or, at a system level, for the co-design or co-production of care.

In the remainder of this section I will explore the idea of medicalisation further and, first, attend to some possible misreadings. To repeat, I do not want to equate medicine and medicalisation. It is possible to have a range of quite different, and more or less expansive, conceptions of medicine. Many doctors are as wary of the possible dangers of reductionism as non-medical critics are. They would simply argue for a less reductionist, more 'holistic' approach to medicine that incorporates what I am calling de-medicalising currents. In other words, many critiques of medicine can also be seen as debates *within* medicine as to its proper character, and there is a long and rich heritage of work by members of the medical profession – for example, in primary care but elsewhere too – that stresses the non-reductionist, collaborative and social dimensions of healthcare.

Nor do I want to suggest that reductionism is inherently bad. The biomedical model cannot simply be seen as some kind of giant mistake. The opposite is nearer the truth. It is partly the huge success and benefits of biomedical thinking that helps to drive medicalisation. Many ill-health phenomena can be successfully classified, treated and resolved by the application of clinical knowledge, including the scientific and technical mindset that accompanies it. Medicalisation is better understood as the over-reaching of the successful biomedical model – as the 'stretching' of the model to arenas, cases or aspects of cases where different models are needed; or as the habitual or presumptive use of a necessarily limited lens on the world.

Finally, we should not assume, and I do not want to imply, that medicalisation is simply 'done by doctors' or is just a product of limited cognitive lenses. There are no doubt occasions when the biomedical model is deliberately and self-consciously advanced by social actors, including doctors. This might occur, for example, in debates about the balance of material in the medical curriculum – where biomedical reductionism still has a prominent place, and many think rightly so. However, in the main, medicalisation happens through underlying social processes – processes which are in many respects unintended. And multiple agents are bound up with these processes – for example, patients, policy makers, corporations, such as pharmaceutical companies – all of whom have some investment in the 'solutions' that biomedical thinking has to offer. This is essentially the same way in which any powerful set of ideas (or ideology or discourse and so on) is socially reproduced and can become institutionally and culturally dominant. Worries about medicalisation are only partly worries about deliberate efforts to promote biomedical thinking (for example, perhaps because it is tied in with specific professional or commercial interests); they are mainly worries about the ways in which underlying models and norms can become 'hard wired' into our institutional and social worlds.

Critiques of 'medicalisation' have been around for about 50 years but they have changed in character over that time. Initially these critiques were largely associated with external critics of the profession of medicine. For example, philosophical and sociological critics of medicine – partly in reaction to positive 'functionalist' accounts of the role of professions as necessary to the maintenance of social order (Parsons, 1951) – were often quite negative about doctors and the power and social advantages they exercised. Influential critics who achieved prominence in the 1970s, such as Ivan Illich and Thomas McKeown, provide a good 'baseline' understanding of (different aspects of) the negative effects of medicalisation.

Ivan Illich, in his celebrated book *Limits to Medicine* (Illich, 1976), argued that the 'ownership' of health by medicine causes multiple problems including the relative 'disablement' and dependency of people who might otherwise take greater responsibility over, and control of, their own health. Illich was also responsible for the widespread dissemination of the concept of 'iatrogenesis', which refers to the ways in which medical intervention can itself cause harm to people. These harms can come about in a variety of ways including side-effects, over-diagnosis and over-treatment (a fact which has more recently become a mainstream concern of policy directed towards healthcare quality improvement).

One of the key worries articulated by Illich, and elaborated in a considerable amount of more recent work in the sociology of health, is that giving undue emphasis to biomedicine adversely alters the nature and quality of our lived experience and social relationships. Things that should be seen as personal, cultural or social matters are translated into medical matters. It is not just 'how we think' but 'what we do' and 'who we are' that is shaped by the biomedical model. Key, and oft-cited, examples here are the medicalisation of birth and death themselves – the concern being that these 'natural' and 'human' processes are remade by being subject to medical perspectives, definitions and social and institutional controls, with the result that people are marginalised (or in some ways even negated) in processes that should be central to their lives and identities. But these worries about the beginning and end of life can be generalised. Critics of medicalisation direct our attention to the multiple ways in which the whole of our lives – including our personal and social identities, as well as our experiences of being 'well' or 'ill' – can be defined (limited and potentially damaged) by biomedical discourses.

Both more temperate in style and more of an insider than Illich, Thomas McKeown is another early figure widely associated with critiquing medicine's claims. In particular McKeown was known for arguing that the battle against infectious diseases (in particular tuberculosis) needed to be understood as a product of economic and social change as well as of medical intervention and that the effects of the latter (for example, of drugs and vaccines) had, compared to the former, been substantially exaggerated. For that reason – although much of the detail and weighting in McKeown's argument remains controversial (Heggie, 2013) – he is often cited as a successful advocate for modern public-health perspectives that apply a broad lens to the social production of health and illness.

McKeown and many subsequent authors thus encourage us to be aware of health services 'over-claiming', of the danger of vested interests being served by these claims and of the risk that seeing health through a predominantly clinical lens results in our collectively missing much else that matters. We are encouraged to open our gaze to other aspects of the social world, including the socioeconomic and material circumstances that directly put people at risk, or protect their health, and that differentially shape life opportunities that also substantially affect health experiences and outcomes. In this respect the broader 'social lens' can be seen as an important corrective to a narrower 'clinical lens'. However, as I will discuss later, there are different ways in which a 'social' or 'public health' outlook can be invoked and operationalised and some of these might be better seen as an extension of medicalisation rather than as a corrective to it. Biomedical discourses are not confined to the clinic – they can spread far and wide. Indeed, recognising this is central to the very idea of medicalisation.

I have highlighted the powerful reductionist tendencies in the biomedical model, but some critics would see this emphasis – given the insights developed by Illich and others – as a rather limited and anodyne account of the nature and implications of medicalisation. They would want to stress the potentially substantial negative effects of reductionist medical tendencies on the experiences and identities of people; and, more broadly, the ways in which medicine embodies and reproduces other forms of social hierarchy (for example, around class, gender and 'race'). Feminist critics of medicalisation, for example, underline the way that medicine 'takes ownership' of areas of women's experience and also reinforces gender hierarchies (for example, through occupational stratification, research agendas and mundane practices).[1]

Without in any way wishing to dissolve these substantive moral and political concerns sociologists have increasingly come to recognise ambivalences and complexities in this area. Indeed, since the 1970s criticisms of medicine have gradually been both qualified (in some cases becoming less stark and oppositional) and extended (applied more broadly beyond clinicians) and have also been absorbed by critically reflexive constituencies within medicine. Specifically, the idea that patients are basically 'victims' of medicalisation is now set against the various ways in which patients not only can be seen to benefit from medicine but also can positively embrace medicine for their own purposes and thereby themselves contribute to processes and forms of medicalisation (Atkinson, 1995; Lupton, 1997). In some respects this is merely one more example of the recognition that the social and policy field is not simply produced and shaped in a 'top-down' way but is a product of agents operating, and pushing against one another, at many levels. This shift from the earliest constructions of medicalisation specifically reflects later currents in sociology. Notably, Deborah Lupton, writing in 1997, showed how Foucauldian readings of medicine both complemented and challenged some of the earlier emphases. This is because Foucault's work famously overturns a conception of power that sees it as exclusively possessed by some specific agents *over* other agents and as necessarily constraining and negative, and proposes a conception in which power is seen as much more widely dispersed and dynamic, and as something that is productive, carrying the potential to make things happen. This kind of reading, which has been extraordinarily influential, does not in any sense diminish the notion that biomedicine is powerful (if anything, it magnifies it), but it shifts the locus of power from specific agents, including doctors, to the circulation of biomedical discourses. In the terms introduced in the last chapter it directs our attention to biomedical ideas as fundamentally powerful building blocks of social practices, habits of mind and institutional organisation.

Medicine beyond medicalisation

As I have emphasised, it is possible, and indeed quite common, for members of the medical profession to place themselves at some critical distance from medicalisation. One reading of this might be that these doctors are self-deluded or practising some more subtle forms of 'false-consciousness'. Even if that were true in some instances, it seems to be an inadequate, and rather glib, way of dealing with the internal complexity of medicine. It is better to start from some recognition of this complexity. We can approach this by using a crude 'three dimensional' model of medicine – medicine as the generator of scientific truths about health, medicine as being about the provision of technological solutions and medicine as a humane profession. It is, roughly speaking, the third dimension – the notion of medicine as a humane profession – that enables doctors to distance themselves from the narrower conception of medicine that is represented in the first two dimensions. Doctors will insist – quite rightly – that medicine is an art as well as a science, and is a human activity as much as a technological one. Medicine, seen from this perspective, does not have to be equated with scientific and technological reductionism.

All professions, and medicine is a paradigm example, can be seen in idealistic terms. Furthermore, it is, I would suggest, a serious mistake to simply dismiss these idealistic constructions. It makes just as much sense to begin by assuming that there is considerable merit in the professional dimension of medicine. The medical profession provides a body of socially recognised experts who bring their knowledge and their humanity, including a preoccupation with both technical and ethical standards, and processes of collective peer scrutiny, to the service of the broader population. It is not only that the three dimensions can fit together neatly, but also that they help to make sense of one another. It is the claim to scientific and technological expertise with regard to health that arguably provides the core rationale for the existence of the profession and helps to justify its pre-eminence in the occupational field of health. But in the exercise of scientific expertise doctors have capacity to treat science as a means to an end and to draw upon other kinds of expertise and wisdom.

According to Freidson (2001), it is precisely this expertise-based and standards-based social influence that gives professionalism its distinctive social role and value. On this account the value of professionalism is that it provides a crucial counter-balance to the social influence of the state and the market. This is not to deny that there is a role for state or market forms of social coordination in the construction or organisation of healthcare – these forms of social coordination can make important contributions (and I will indicate this more fully in Chapters Three and Four). It is, rather, that the 'logics' underpinning these modes of social coordination need to be complemented by what Freidson labels as the logic of professionalism. It is the latter that not only helps to insulate practices from the hazards both of bureaucracy and market forces but also underpins the possibility of knowledgeable responsiveness to variations between individuals, their trajectories and personal and social contexts. Good healthcare needs the logic of professionalism – not only in the case of doctors but for all the other constitutive occupational groups – to form a core part of its underlying rationale or foundational architecture. Of course each of what I have called the three dimensions of medicine can be viewed as problematic; but all of these criticisms can, at least to some extent, be incorporated into a revised or enlarged vision of medical professionalism.

The scientific–technological basis of medicine can, for example, be criticised as 'partially sighted'. One familiar line of criticism is that scientific claims can easily be over-simplified and over-stated – that legitimate disputes *within* science can be underplayed or that claims that have validity in connection with a specific range of cases are being applied to cases where they lack validity (such as drugs that have tested efficacy for a specific population or treatment group but not necessarily others). But a deeper line of criticism focuses on the *inherent limitations* of scientific knowledge. Scientific knowledge cannot provide all of the knowledge and understanding needed to inform healthcare – because, for example, the experiences and meanings of ill-health cannot be adequately 'captured' by a scientific orientation. The experiences and circumstances of people – who are facing the uncertainty, emotional disruption and existential disequilibrium produced by either physical or mental ill-health – call for other forms of knowledge. For example, they call for listening, insight and understanding, along with practical support with the challenges of adapting to what can feel like a whole new life-world for such people. The same concern attaches to a technological mindset. Not everything is amenable to being 'fixed'. This is notoriously the case in relation to death itself. But, of course, the same is true for the rest of life – the instabilities, threats and suffering encountered throughout life (because of illness and much else besides) cannot all be technologically managed. Other forms of response are needed, and defensible forms of healthcare professionalism will need a broad-based repertoire of responses.

As well as recognising the limits of technological thinking, critics can point to the risks and costs of medicine as technology. I will not say more here about the substantial question of iatrogenesis, including the potential social and human costs of the societal over-dependence on 'fixes'– think, for example, of the debates about the right balance between approaching people's 'over-eating' through tablets or surgery and approaching it through other avenues such as peer support and informal education. However, it is important to mention the huge financial costs of a highly technological approach to healthcare. The cost of healthcare, of which the costs of purchasing, supporting and using technology are a substantial part, has become a major political and economic issue in high-income countries. (I will come back to this in the next section of the chapter.)

The third dimension of medicine – medicine as humane profession – is, clearly, not exempt from criticism. The central concern here is the threat of professional domination. Although the 'packaging' of professionalism might make a feature of the language of service, the substance, critics argue, is the relative control of clients for the advancement of the economic and social status of members of the professional group. This is the way, critics suggest, that the ideology of professionalism works. These kinds of criticisms are long standing, cannot be easily be dismissed and have been well recognised by doctors and other health professionals. Indeed there have been multiple efforts to try to respond to them and this is one of the reasons why ideas such as 'partnership working' or 'shared decision making' have come to prominence in recent health policy.

The three dimensions of medicine intersect in many different configurations, producing multiple 'medicines'. The result is that there are no clearly agreed boundaries to medicine and very many vantage points that one can adopt from 'inside' medicine. For example, there is a tendency for the professional–client model that informs medicine as humane profession to reinforce, through its core place in clinical medicine, a somewhat individual-oriented and response-oriented version of medicine. However, there are also important strands in medicine that emphasise population-oriented and prevention-oriented perspectives and frame science and technology less through an interest in individual bodies and more through an interest in the constitution of the 'social body'. In this case what has sometimes been called 'social medicine' can stand in opposition to 'individualised medicine', just as 'humanistic medicine' will sometimes define itself in distinction to 'scientific medicine'.

It should be noted that the defence of a more holistic professional role for doctors against the criticism of scientific–technological reductionism can be matched by a possible defence of the value of biomedicine separated from the danger of medical professional domination. (On the latter analysis it is the third dimension of medicine that can carry the real danger and not the more 'neutral' first two dimensions of science and technology.) Such separation might be achieved in part by reconfiguring professionalism and building more 'equal' partnership-based ways of working (as just alluded to above). But it might be accomplished at a more fundamental level by the 'liberation' of biomedical knowledge from the professional sphere – through the widest possible dissemination of biomedical knowledge, technology and practice.

Hence, for every criticism of medicine there is a possible defence of medicine. Doctors and others can attempt to show why specific criticisms are mistaken, or, to the extent that they believe criticisms have substance, they can try to reform medical cultures and practices so that the force of criticisms comes to have less relevance and purchase. The currents within medicine are not only multifarious but are constantly adapting and evolving. In other words, the cases that can be made for de-medicalisation can also invariably be interpreted as cases for 're-medicalisation', that is, for revising or extending approaches to medicine. The reasons for the resilience and adaptability of medicine are not just negative ones – it is not merely about the medical profession 'clinging on' to their social influence. Rather, to echo earlier remarks, it has to be conceded that medicine contributes something valuable even in its narrowest forms – a reductionist 'fix' is not everything, but ask all those people who have benefited from medical intervention and they will no doubt insist that it is still a great deal.

Nonetheless, there are very many people who think that the prevailing version of medicine is still dominated by an overly narrow biomedical model, in a way that does a disservice to healthcare and the promotion of health more generally. It may be that the possibilities of medicine are very broad, but the worry is that the present configurations of medicine and healthcare are out of balance. In what follows I will summarise some of the arguments for claiming that this imbalance exists and their implications for rethinking health policy. I will then go on to introduce some of the possible responses – which I am loosely classifying as de-medicalising responses, or as calls for more person-centred healthcare. Although I think these responses are fundamentally important, I should make it clear from the outset that they are not themselves unproblematic and the following chapters seek to open up some of the tensions within, and potential limitations of, 'person-centred' models of care in the same way that this one has for biomedical models.

Health policy out of kilter and medicine out of control?

It is not particularly controversial to say that health policy in high-income countries is out of kilter – is, in other words, in some important respects unbalanced and dysfunctional. This is a position adopted by many commentators, and is implicit in the various reforming currents that have arisen within mainstream policy circles. The relevant imbalances can be described in different genres and in different terms, and in this section I will illustrate them by drawing on sceptical voices from both outside and inside of healthcare. Some of what they have in common can be summarised very simply: that healthcare expenditure is often wasted or spent on the wrong things.

The distinguished ethicist Daniel Callahan has set out one systematic account of imbalances in his analysis of, and calls for a reorientation of, US healthcare. For example, in *Taming the Beloved Beast* (2009) he overtly focused on the escalating costs of medical technology but, in so doing, he made a passionate (and carefully argued) call for changing the philosophical centre of gravity of healthcare. The book's 'headline message' – which can be read as a political wake-up call – is conveyed in its sub-title, *How Medical Technology Costs Are Destroying Our Health Care System*. This can be interpreted on one level as a complaint purely about waste, inefficiency or financial sustainability. But, although these financial concerns are of critical importance, the complaint is much deeper.

For example, Callahan takes a cold, hard look at the fact that a great deal of healthcare expenditure and effort serves to make no more than marginal improvements (and possibly even no difference or a negative difference) to the health experiences of some individuals (sometimes only a few individuals), while at the same time the basic needs of many others are neglected. Callahan argues that what is needed is a 'cultural revolution' to overturn and replace the organising values of American healthcare:

> We have a culture addicted to the idea of unlimited progress and the technological innovation that is its natural child ... In its present form, this is an unsustainable value. There must be limits. American healthcare is radically American: individualistic, scientifically ambitious, market intoxicated, suspicious of government, and profit driven ... The medical model that needs change encompasses a combination of Manichean and utopian values: that suffering of any kind, but mainly biological suffering, is an inherent evil; that death is intrinsically wrong and should be the main enemy of medicine ... And that endless medical progress should be pursued. There is, many seem to believe, no such thing as enough good health. These are understandable values, the Enlightenment played out in medicine. They have become, however, the wrong ones to undergird healthcare systems and the practice of medicine that aims for equitable access, a good balance between health and other social needs, and

that are affordable, sustainable in the long run, and accessible to all. (Callahan, 2009, p 7)

Callahan is particularly critical of the individualism that frames much of the US system and argues for purposes and priorities to be defined against a conception of the 'common good' – that is, a notion of what is good for the health and well-being of society as a whole and what it is reasonable for 'average' individuals to expect, rather than for a few to be able to 'buy' – that is, for significant attention to be given to equality and solidarity. Some parts of Callahan's thesis are much more contentious than others. For example, his overall championing of a health economy that has a different organisational rationality, with a changed balance of market and government coordination – that is, is in broad terms, more like a European approach – would obviously not go down well in all quarters of the USA. But, in considerably less 'populist' terms even than that, he is prepared to follow the logic of his argument and address the issue of which valuable things might not get done or provided, following his 'revolution'. In this respect he is an exceptionally scrupulous and responsible commentator and one who serves as an exemplar for the core concern of this book – that any 'rebalancing' will involve 'costs' because we cannot have everything in life or in health policy.

In particular, Callahan is prepared to underline the implications of his case for a check on unbridled individualism in healthcare. If the health system is to be reformed so as to serve the overall good, then this means that there are limits to how far individuals can expect 'boutique' provision for themselves:

> What might be of immense value to us as individuals may not be compatible with an equitable healthcare system, aiming for a common good, not just the private good. (Callahan, 2009, p 2)

However, large parts of Callahan's case are not highly contentious but coincide with widely held concerns about, and very orthodox analyses of, the wastefulness of much expensive healthcare provision. There is, for example, now a substantial and highly respected body of work on the risks and costs of over-treatment, which I will discuss below. More broadly it is worth noting that the two 'registers' that are combined in Callahan's account – of financial expense and waste, on the one hand, and of philosophical shortcomings, on the other, are often linked together – although sometimes less explicitly. For example, it is quite common for reforms aimed at service improvement for good-quality care to be bound in with discourses about improving productivity or financial efficiency.

Many of the same factors that produce the seeming imperative to treat and the risks, and waste, of over-treatment also produce some of the other suggested imbalances in health policy – for example, the pervasive problem that health systems tend to be more responsive to the demands of the better-off rather than to the needs of the worse-off. Different analysts will look in slightly different directions for the explanations. Critics of the medical profession, or of biomedical discourses more widely, will stress the power of narrow biomedical norms in defining what count as problems and solutions within health systems. Critics of the state and the growth of bureaucratic rationality, or healthcare 'managerialism' in both private and public sectors, will underline the rigidities of institutional norms that govern success. Critics of markets will point to the effect of private corporations 'pushing' various kinds of medical technology and to the consequences of various degrees of marketisation in healthcare (even within single-payer systems) that tend towards constructing healthcare as a commodity and measuring success in terms of productivity or 'output' – whether or not the latter means 'profit' or simply high performance levels in competitive/comparative market cultures and systems. I am not pursuing an explanatory agenda here, but it seems sensible to be alive to all these possibilities. But each of these readings arguably points to relatively surface features in comparison to those that Callahan is stressing – namely, the worry that the health system is based on the wrong underlying assumptions and purposes, and that what is needed is an alternative conception of healthcare. For many commentators a growing worry is that the deficits of the US system identified here – as a highly market-led and unequal one that does not feature solidarity as an organising idea – are 'spreading' across the globe as part of the ascendancy of a neoliberal political economy (Mooney, 2012).

Any full account of the perceived ills of historically dominant philosophical and policy tendencies – such as Callahan's concerns about the escalating influence of the technological mindset – has to be set in the context of socio-political debates about global and local markets and the commercialisation of healthcare. But it is worth underlining that the technological mindset is already built into the logic of the biomedical model, and noting how this has produced what has come to be widely accepted as a largely 'common sense' extension of the spheres and practices of medicalisation. For example, Pereira Gray and colleagues (2016) have argued that the scale of medicalisation has mushroomed over what they describe as 'a single professional lifetime', with general medical practice having 'reversed from being mainly reactive work with doctors responding to patients' symptoms, to a pro-active mass assessment of risk with extensive issuing of treatments, increasingly for people without symptoms at all' (Pereira Gray et al, 2016, p 7). In addition to the mass prescribing of statins to help prevent cardiovascular disease, they cite other examples – programmes of mass immunisation and mass screening, with the lowering of thresholds for intervention (for example, for hypertension, prediabetes and anxiety and depression). This shift shows how the central orientation of the biomedical model – towards disease management and treatment – can be very elastic in application as our conceptions of, and approaches to, such management or treatment evolve.

Pereira Gray et al also echo many of the points already made in this chapter – in particular they stress the convergence of medical and social science attitudes towards medicalisation, with each 'side' increasingly developing a more balanced account of the harms and benefits of medicine, and a greater recognition of the contribution of multiple parties – including patients – to the production of medicalisation. They acknowledge, for example, the contribution of market and commercial interests, the rise of new technological modes and sectors (such as biotechnology), the interests and professionalisation of doctors, but also the activity of patients and publics both in challenging and in furthering medicalisation – including through the huge consumption of 'over-the-counter' medicines. They also note how this extension of medicalisation at a population level is underpinned, but also 'driven', by system-level developments, including the integration of information technology into health services, that enable and increasingly 'require' the monitoring of populations according to evolving conceptions of risk. This account of the 'massification' of medicalisation shows how the equation of the clinical realm with the individual doctor–patient relationship or with small-scale spaces is mistaken. The shift to the social perspective or to broader 'public health' considerations can be one response to the narrowness of medicalisation, but it can equally be another avenue for extending medicalisation.

In recent years there has been a significant level of convergence between social and philosophical critiques of medicalisation and mainstream concerns within health services and quality-improvement research. The concern that there is the growing risk of, and in some areas the reality of, 'too much medicine' has been recognised by editorials and conferences hosted by the *BMJ* and other influential medical bodies. It is important to acknowledge that somewhat different points are being made by various contributors to this field, but nonetheless these coalesce around the broad ideas of 'too much medicine' and/or 'over-diagnosis'. Carter et al (2015) usefully distinguish between the former as 'broad' and useful for policy advocacy and the latter as being more amenable to a range of more technical definitions, depending upon specific purposes.

There are many parallels between the critical concerns aired from outside medicine and mainstream analyses. For example, a very important tradition of health-services research has focused on 'practice variations' within health systems. This work begins by mapping differences in service provision, for example, the number of a certain kind of investigative or treatment procedures in different geographical parts of the system. But it then goes on to ask a number of more analytical questions – specifically, (a) what accounts for these practice variations, for example, how far are they explained by differences in the health needs of the local population or by the characteristics of the providers? (b) if we factor out differences between the health profiles of populations what differences do these practice variations make to health outcomes and experiences? In plain terms, does the provision of more treatments always mean better healthcare? This research shows that the answer to this question is 'no'. Jack Wennberg is the researcher who pioneered this line of enquiry and he has looked, for example, at outcome data related to patients admitted to hospital with hip fractures, heart attacks and colon cancer who received higher and lower intensities of care simply as a product of where they were treated, showing that patients with a 'high intensity' of interventions had on average worse or no better outcomes (Wennberg, 2010). In other words, there are now well-documented examples of 'unproductive' health provision.

The high-profile evidence-based medicine movement was fuelled in significant part by this kind of research. It has forced home the question of how we know whether interventions 'work' and has fed into an increased level of 'informed scepticism' about the automatic value of clinical intervention on the part of professionals and publics alike. Over time this movement ought to mean that the risk of over-treatment is reduced. But this is far from an easy matter and it is important to appreciate that there are significant pressures – as highlighted by Callahan – that push in the direction of over-treatment.

The notion of over-treatment is, of course, not straightforward and involves both empirical and value judgements. Recognising over-treatment involves something like an assessment that there are no or few significant benefits from an intervention, such that risks or positive harms exceed potential benefits. This may be obvious in clear-cut cases of iatrogenesis – where the direct harms caused by clinical intervention obviously overshadow the hoped-for benefits – for example, because procedures frequently go badly wrong or drugs have very serious short- or long-term side-effects – but it can extend much more widely. And the presence of harm is not always so evident. The most well-known example of over-prescribing, for example, is the over-use of antibiotics. In many cases there is no question of significant levels of immediate harm being caused to the individuals getting the individual prescription. However, there is a very substantial and longer-term level of harm threatened to the whole world population if excess prescription of antibiotics is not checked. This can serve as an analogy for some of the complications of specifying over-treatment – we need to be ready to look at system-level effects and costs as well as immediate risks to individuals. As is well known with antibiotics, some treatments will make no difference to individual outcomes, some may do more direct harm than good (for example, because of allergic reactions), but even those that are harmless or better at an individual level may be undesirable because of their collective effects.

One of the factors raising both the quantity and the profile of over-treatment is the considerably expanded potential for diagnosis, including 'over diagnosis' in one sense or another. Modern medicine has seen both a proliferation of diagnostic technologies and a huge growth in the opportunities for and routinisation of health monitoring. While in many respects clinical monitoring is a boon, and arguably a welcome feature of the greater incorporation of a preventive perspective into clinical medicine, it has at the same time generated new kinds of practical and ethical problems. These are familiar, for example, as well-known problems facing population-screening programmes: what are the social and psychological costs not only of 'false positives' but of validly labelling people as 'at risk' in certain respects? Even more specifically, under what circumstances do the identification of risk factors and the practical possibility of intervention make such screening of measurable clinical benefit to individuals and communities? The concern that specific screening programmes do not always successfully address these challenges or meet the thresholds necessary to be of net benefit is fast becoming a concern of much more general relevance. As with population screening, the medical monitoring gaze is often focused on people who are basically asymptomatic or, at least, is capable of picking up indicators of risk that are unrelated to any symptoms that have been presented. This also means that doctors, and the lens of diagnosis, are often directed not at diseases per se, but at pre-disease states or biomedical markers of possible disease. There is a fairly evident worry here of constantly multiplying the disease-like entities in the world and of pathologising a good deal of normal biological variation.

Here again there is a clear correspondence between those ideological critics of medicine who have warned against the definition of various 'life problems' through clinical categories and the more precise worries that have been rehearsed by those within medicine who have identified over-diagnosis as a growing problem that needs to be checked. The *BMJ* editorial 'Too much medicine; too little care', authored by Paul Glasziou and colleagues (2013), identified 'Signs of overdiagnosis':

> 'Red flags' for possible overdiagnosis
> The incidence is increasing while mortality stays the same
> Labelling of a risk factor or biomarker to sound like a disease
> Shift in diagnostic definitions or thresholds with no clear evidence that benefits are greater than harms.

The authors offer examples of over-diagnosis, including the tripling in the incidence of thyroid cancer in the USA, Australia and elsewhere between 1975 and 2012 unaccompanied by any change in the death rate. They suggest that this is best described as an 'epidemic of diagnosis' rather than a true rise in cancer incidence. They also argue that small changes in disease definitions, which redraw the boundaries between normal and abnormal, have greatly expanded the proportion of the population with disease labels, and cite hypertension, diabetes, osteoporosis, high cholesterol, obesity and cognitive impairment as examples. They argue:

> A growing frustration in clinical medicine is that we are now so busy managing the proliferation of risk factors, 'incidentalomas', and the worried well that we lack the time to care properly for those who are seriously ill. As the definitions of common conditions such as diabetes and kidney disease have expanded and the categories and boundaries of mental disorders have grown, our time and attention for the most worryingly ill, disturbed, and vulnerable patients has shrunk. Too much medicine is harming both the sick and well ... With the economic crisis and the challenge of providing universal care for all, it's time to find ways to safely and fairly wind back the harms of too much medicine.

Of course it may be that other researchers would question the merits of some of the examples cited by these authors or others in the growing community of 'over-diagnosis' researchers, but that is not the core issue. These researchers are helping to articulate and specify a very important concern, namely, that even if measured purely on its own terms medicine does not always succeed and that there is a need to pay attention to why that is and how thresholds for intervention should be set so as to reduce that risk.

Another crucially important, and potentially hidden, complication of assessing the value of diagnoses and the effectiveness of treatments is the difficulty of determining the relative benefit of interventions to specific individuals. I will say more about this in the next few chapters but it is too important a theme to ignore here. Outside of a narrow biomedical perspective, interventions do not have a fixed, 'objective' or person-independent value. Different things matter to different people – depending upon their histories, circumstances, life projects and preferences. Take the case of hormone replacement therapy, for example. Leaving aside the very general arguments about its costs and benefits and, for example, different, and sometimes competing, feminist readings of its value, there is no good reason why two individual women who are (hypothetically) in the same clinical situation – facing what are defined as the same symptoms, risks and benefits – should not have different preferences about treatment. They may well weigh the risks and benefits differently, indeed they may even each construct some things primarily as 'risks' that the other one constructs as benefits and vice versa (Komesaroff and Rothfield, 1997). The same is potentially true for all interventions – some factors that will be salient or central to specific individuals will be marginal or irrelevant for others. This means that any measure of effectiveness or output that is based on generalised assumptions about interventions 'working', or being 'evidence based', can be over-simplistic and can actually mask important clinical failures (as a result of what Mulley et al (2012b) call 'preference mis-diagnosis'). There are a number of studies that have shown how services – in many areas including coronary heart disease, prostate disease, abnormal menstrual bleeding and so on – that were properly responsive to the informed choices of individuals, rather than the perceptions of clinicians about appropriate care, would have resulted in lower levels of clinical intervention (Mulley et al, 2012a).

In short, there are many credible voices, ranging from critical commentators to mainstream researchers and practitioners within healthcare, who agree that much of current healthcare is neither effective nor equitable. This applies even if we take the most conventional and restricted readings of what counts as being effective and equitable, that is, delivering clinical interventions where they lead to better clinical outcomes, and where the interventions are directed at people who will benefit from them, and are not wasted by being misdirected or by being ineffective or harmful. But in the process of articulating these concerns these voices also help to raise questions about what can and should count as effective or equitable in healthcare. For example, the fact that treatments can be ('equally') delivered to people who do not want or value them suggests that our yardsticks of both effectiveness and equity need to be recalibrated in a way that reflects people's personal circumstances and preferences. The emphasis in the 'too much medicine' literature is thus on ensuring that individuals who are being offered healthcare can reasonably be judged to have benefited and not been harmed by the offer; but there is also enough discussion of marshalling resources fairly to provide clear echoes of Dan Callahan's contention (cited above) that healthcare needs to be judged by its contribution to the 'common good' and not merely as a 'private good'.

Re-balancing health policy: introducing person-centredness

There is a continuous search for a more balanced approach to health policy. This is both reflected in and furthered by what I have described as the philosophical transition. Politicians, patient organisations and other commentators regularly cite changing circumstances and call for further reforms to health services and public health policies. Many of these calls can be seen as the 'mirror image' of the critiques of the biomedical model reviewed above and, specifically, of a reductionist presumption in health policy that 'over-concentrates' on bodies (rather than whole persons), the management of diseases or disease risks (rather than the promotion of health or support of well-being), scientific–technical thinking (with the potential neglect of broader forms of knowledge and understanding) and professional authority (rather than partnership or dispersed agency). These calls, in different ways, involve either partly displacing or at least complementing the influence of a narrow biomedical model by the adoption of broader models that I am summarising as 'person-centred'. Here person-centredness is not used just in the restricted sense mentioned at the beginning of the chapter, where it relates to practices that 'suit' persons, but in an extended sense in which person-centred policies and services also 'connect with', engage with and are responsive to people, including to their projects, preferences and participation.

We do not have to see these rebalancing or reform efforts as a consequence of the failure of the biomedical model. Some of them might be presented as a consequence of its success. Once the daily threat of dying from infectious diseases, and the impact of many diseases on the length or quality of life, has been substantially reduced – as has happened in affluent health economies – it becomes necessary to look elsewhere to further enhance provision. This, it might be argued, reflects an ascent up Maslow's famous 'hierarchy of needs'. But while some reforms can be seen as complementing existing health-service provision others are clearly about changing its character. And in both cases the changes that are being called for are not all confined to rarefied concerns (at the top of the hierarchy of needs) but relate to indisputably basic goods including life and death. This is most clearly the case for some important complementary currents – such as for 'health promotion' – where a strong emphasis is often given to preventive agendas, and where measures designed to tackle tobacco smoking and other 'life-style' factors or well-being determinants such as social isolation, for example, are often justified in large measure by their intended effects on both mortality and morbidity. The changing patterns of smoking, for example, brought about to some extent by deliberate educational, cultural and regulatory change, are as relevant to life saving and life extension as the most 'high tech' surgical advances. But analogous changes in clinical climates, including educational and communication reforms, are needed just as much and have equally important implications.

Just as smoking can kill you or, as the warning puts it, 'seriously damage your health', so too can poor health-service relationships. As just noted in connection with the problem of 'preference mis-diagnosis', there is no point in having even the best 'clinical solutions' in place if they are misdirected or deployed inappropriately or ineffectively because of a lack of proper 'connection' between professionals and patients. A high-profile and incredibly wasteful example of this is sometimes referred to as the problem of 'non-compliance' (often now described using the language of 'adherence' or even 'concordance') (Horne et al, 2005). This occurs when doctors or other professionals prescribe medicines but patients do not take them or do not take them in the way the prescriber intends. There can be many reasons for this – for example, the patient may actively not want to take them (a case of preference mis-diagnosis); the life circumstances of the patient or their personal habits may make it difficult to take them; or there may simply be a failure to understand or internalise the significance of the medicines or the 'instructions' that go with them. The effect of each of these things might be reduced or eliminated by better communication. In some cases, if the right form and level of communication (and practical support) are in place this could result in substantial health implications (as well as better resource use). But these points about the need to change climates within health services and the importance of successful 'connection' between professionals and patients, or more broadly between the 'clinical realm' and the 'social realm', do not only apply to the proper use of medicines but to the full gamut of ways in which services can make a difference in people's lives.

In other words, engaging effectively with, and working with, patients and populations is a critical dimension of health-policy reform, and one that has the potential to impact on conventional indicators of policy success – mortality and morbidity outcomes and cost-effectiveness. But the rationale for such engagement also springs from deeper and wider sources. This rationale is sometimes expressed in the language of ethics – relating to people properly requires us to treat them with respect and to recognise, and be responsive to, their identities and autonomy. In so far as we choose to talk in terms of purposes or 'outcomes', then the impetus here is to address concerns closer to the top of the hierarchy of needs, that is, to help meet people's needs for meaningful relationships and for self-actualisation. Although they are less 'basic', the needs at the top of the hierarchy are just as important as, and sometimes more important than, those at the bottom. This can be seen, for instance, in circumstances where an individual chooses some other end over life prolongation (for example, not to suffer the costs and risks of further treatment where this compromises their ability to complete some project that is important to them). The presumption in healthcare ethics would be to respect such a preference and to see it as an important sign of respect for the person and their values. To try to prolong their life by unwanted treatment when this is not the most important thing from their point of view would be seen as simply wrong. The hierarchy of value here – between survival and self-actualisation – is not straightforward.

As I am indicating, there is no singular coherent counter-weight to the influence of the biomedical model in health policy. There are various anti-reductionist tendencies that, for the sake of simplicity, I have labelled as 'person-centred' tendencies. Advocating for healthcare to be more 'person-centred' can be understood as a call for an alternative set of 'organising ideas' for healthcare to the ideas that cluster around the biomedical model. This, albeit crude, shorthand is arguably defensible, because many of the elements of anti-reductionism can be traced back to a shift of emphasis from 'diseased bodies' to 'persons'. Of course the suggestion here is not that in being responsive to persons, health services should stop being responsive to diseases; rather, it is that the latter needs to be placed in the context of the former in ways that both extend and modify our fundamental conceptions of healthcare. As indicated in Chapter One, this transition is about attending to all of the ways that clinical concerns are nested within social concerns. Ultimately the thought here is not that better healthcare literally equates to healthcare which people experience fewer medical interventions and take fewer medicines (although, as discussed, that will be true some of the time) but to healthcare in which the biomedical model is much less influential in defining the overall shape of healthcare.

Attending to 'persons' draws much into the frame that otherwise might fall outside of it. Indeed it might be said that the healthcare agenda not only expands but 'explodes' when we shift our attention in this way. In the remainder of this section I can just indicate some of the dimensions of this explosion. I suggest that appeals to be 'person-centred' can usefully be seen as summoning up four overlapping dimensions of persons: *persons as agents, persons as suffering, persons as multi-layered* and *persons as relational*.

First, as just highlighted, attending to persons includes responding to their 'choices', preferences and values. We need to be ready to relate to people as agents, as at least partly responsible for shaping what happens in their lives and as entitled to be party to decisions that affect them. This idea has, of course, come to be accepted as a central norm of defensible healthcare through the language of 'respect for autonomy'. Indeed this recognition of agency and autonomy is perhaps the most common way in which healthcare cultures have come to acknowledge the crucial distinction between the treatment of bodies and persons.

But there is more to persons than their agency and autonomy. Even starting from the case of an individual who is suffering from a disease, the change of emphasis directs our attention to the suffering as well as the disease – to the experience of illness within individual people's lives and to all the challenges of understanding, connecting to, engaging with and supporting people both in their common capacity for suffering and in their individual distinctiveness. Thinking about persons means considering dimensions that extend beyond those that attach to bodies. This, in turn, requires us to attach weight to different kinds of practices and different forms of knowledge.

When we make persons our focus we are reminded that they have an internal complexity and depth – every individual is multi-layered. This layering can be captured in different kinds of language – for example, in addition to talking about their beliefs and preferences (as well as their biological make-up) we might talk about their emotional lives and/or their psychological resilience or their unconscious and so on. One aspect of this 'layering' is that people have a 'self-understanding' that underpins and informs their autonomy – they have the capacity to partly 'stand outside' and reflect on their own complex constitution, their multi-layered nature and their personal histories and future-oriented projects.

In addition, and crucially, people can be only very partially understood in individual terms. Persons are fundamentally *relational* – that is, they are constituted in relationship with one another and with groups of persons. People have shared histories that form them both causally and in terms of common frameworks of meaning and identity – they grow up with families and friends and within social contexts and their (unique) identities, hopes and plans are bound up with those of the communities and institutions in which they live and work and that provide them with both opportunities and constraints. If we – whether as a health professional or a lay person – want to help someone it will often be important, and sometimes essential, to have insight into these facts about individual and social constitution – who is this person, what has shaped them and is shaping them, what matters to them and what is possible for them, given their circumstances? Part of attending to these questions, for example, is to appreciate that people's preferences about clinical outcomes will typically be integrated with concerns about, and constraints upon, other aspects of their well-being, identity and projects.

This broad interpretation of person-centredness thus transcends a purely individualist conception of persons. To attend to persons entails thinking both about individuality and social bonds. It also means embracing various kinds of plurality: people are obviously many in number, and diverse. Everything that is relevant to an individual person is multiplied many times – individuals and groups may choose to exercise their agency in contrasting ways, making contributions and demands that push policies and provision in different directions. (The balances between individually oriented and community-/population-oriented emphases within the 'social turn' are a theme that will recur in the following chapters.)

I have outlined these features of person-centred thinking in abstract terms – as aspects of a changing cultural field. But, of course, for individual actors (health professionals, lay people and so on) incorporating these features into their ways of seeing and thinking will often involve personal change – often including a bundle of potential 'gestalt switches'. For example, for a professional to fully see their patients as partners, or for a patient to be comfortable thinking of themselves as responsible for their own health or as a potential policy actor, is not always an easy matter.

Conclusion

The dimensions of personhood that I have pointed towards – persons as agents, persons as having a capacity for suffering that calls forth a response, persons as complex, multi-layered individuals, and persons as social or relational – need to be understood in combinations and in relation to one another. Any tendency to highlight one and neglect the others is liable to fail to do justice to personhood. Attending to these dimensions is not just relevant in the 'clinical moment', for example, for understanding what determines a good consultation. It is of fundamental importance to the whole field of health and social policy. If we move away from the consultation and sweep back in time or scale to consider, for example, the social determinants of health and well-being, then we need to think about persons and not just bodies. Of course there are very important issues to investigate about physical causation but this is bound up with the investigation of culture and agency. A prevention agenda, let alone a broader health-promotion agenda, will not get very far unless it engages with the life-worlds, values and priorities, resources and capacities of individuals or populations. The same is true if we look forward in time, for example, to imagine new models of health-related organisation. If organisations are to be suited to, and responsive to, persons, then they need to be designed with all of these dimensions in mind.

In this chapter I have presented a simple four-dimensional picture of personhood for the purpose of giving substance to the idea and challenge of 'person-centred' healthcare. I am not particularly interested in advocating for my four-dimensional picture (rather, I take it for granted that it will have both strengths and weaknesses compared to other accounts). However, I do want to insist that it is important to recognise the multi-dimensionality of persons – including the inherent complications and tensions this generates – if we are to seriously invoke person-centredness as a guide to policy.

Reforms are being approached here as entailing various kinds of rebalancing, and specifically as about finding new organising ideas or foundational DNA for health policy. There is no easy way to accomplish this rebalancing or, in other words, to complete the philosophical transition that is underway. Framing health services around a biomedical model produces problems – as we have seen – but it also has some serious advantages. The reductionist emphasis helps to circumscribe the relevant range of considerations. The more we resist the reductionism, the more things, by definition, open up. A healthcare system that is responsive to persons – in their individual complexity and social constitution and relatedness – is one that has to think and act much more expansively. Its architects and agents – who, by definition, become much more numerous, will have to coordinate their efforts while being pushed and pulled in multiple directions, and will inevitably find that they are wrestling with very many competing and conflicting demands. I will explore both the importance and the challenges of rebalancing healthcare – from 'medicine' to 'persons' – in more depth in the next three chapters. As I have just noted, I do not think it makes sense to practically 'split apart' the dimensions of personhood, but I will frame these three chapters around different possible emphases – people acting as choosers (while also needing to be cared for); people seen 'holistically' (in terms of both their 'inner' and 'social' constitution); and people in their uniqueness or (relative) distinctiveness from one another.

Note

[1] See, for example, White (2016).

THREE

Choosing care

Ella and Grant have just moved into the area and are looking for a primary care health centre to use. They look on the web and ask neighbours and colleagues for advice. One big factor for them is their work schedules, which make it extremely difficult to attend appointments except in the evenings. They are looking for a centre that offers an extensive range of evening services and appointments and that does not seem to have attracted any significant official or unofficial criticisms. In the end this makes their choice relatively easy.

Stefan sees his primary care doctor about an itchy skin patch he has developed on his leg. He has ignored it for a few weeks but has started to worry about it and decided he needs to get it checked out. His doctor says 'I'm not sure what it is but I'm pretty sure it's nothing too serious. I suggest you keep an eye on it for another couple of weeks and see if it settles down but, if you like, I will refer you to a specialist dermatologist straight away. We can do either thing. It's up to you.'

Anya comes away from the meeting she and her husband have had with the care team with a very heavy heart. There is the possibility of another round of chemotherapy. The team are proposing it but they are making cautious claims about its likely effectiveness. On balance they think it should protect and extend her life and that is why they are suggesting it. But, obviously, it is up to her and her family to make the decision to go ahead. The situation seems completely hopeless to her, and further intervention feels pointless, but then she knows how worn and weary she is. Perhaps she is not thinking straight. The local doctor she trusts most is visiting this evening – they will all have to think about it together.

One of the concerns, rehearsed in the previous chapter, about a strongly biomedical model of healthcare was the danger of a concentration of power in the hands of professionals. A key policy response to this concern is to focus on strengthening the role of others, especially patients and patients' families or carers. The overarching worry is that healthcare is seen too much as a product of professional or system-level agency and that the agency of patients and publics is not properly recognised or drawn upon. In part, this agenda can be seen as about 'correcting' or compensating for unwarranted hierarchies with an aspiration towards greater equality of respect and influence. At the level of the individual clinical encounter this is sometimes expressed in the call for a shift away from a paternalistic professional–client relationship to a relationship in which the client has more involvement and 'say' – a more balanced or 'equal' relationship, or one based upon a professional–client 'partnership'. But this kind of rationale can be seen as but one feature of a much broader social landscape in which individuals expect to be able to make decisions for themselves. This applies not only to countless kinds of 'consumer' practices but also, more fundamentally, to the core norms of liberal and market-oriented societies, in which being able to shape one's own life, and at root to define and shape oneself, is widely taken for granted as a basic good. Another related rationale – which also has parallels with a key defence of liberalism – is about the freeing up and harnessing of human resource – including people's motivation, energy and relevant expertise – so as to make available more 'person power' and relevant intelligence to the health system.

The potential implications of rethinking agency in health systems are substantial and diverse. Once we start seeing and treating people as healthcare actors – as having something to contribute to their own care and to health systems and environments – many possibilities emerge. Some of these are already absorbed into mainstream thinking and others are more challenging or radical, and are often realised only in pockets or at the margins of systems. The former includes the expectation that patients should play an active role in clinical decision making that affects them. The latter extend much more widely – questioning why 'lay people' are often allowed to be influential only in circumscribed instances (such as in relation to participation in their own clinical care conversations or even 'self-care'), when their agency and perspectives could be equally influential in agenda setting and design decisions in all aspects of service planning, care provision, research, resource allocation and so on. In other words, why should they be allowed only to play specific pre-defined games according to other people's rules, when they should be deciding on the games and rules themselves? This question highlights the potential to move beyond an individualist or consumerist conception of agency and towards more civic, social and democratic conceptions of social action. I will come back to this thought in a few places in what follows, and particularly in the final chapter of this book. In this chapter I will be concentrating on the some of the more mainstream and circumscribed examples of rethinking agency. This emphasis is not meant in any way to question the importance of more radical aspirations, but merely to underline both the positive case for, and some of the complications of, currents of thought that are already widely accepted.

'Choice' can be used as one form of shorthand for this mainstream agenda. I will adopt this shorthand for now as way of proceeding but, as already noted, approaches to recognising and harnessing agency take a variety of forms, use a variety of terms and have different potential implications.

Shared decision making and evidence-based patient choice

The idea of shared decision making (SDM) has, in recent years, been widely advocated by policy makers and has been accepted by many as an important professional ideal, although it is still far from being a professional norm in practice (Coulter and Collins, 2011; Coulter, 2016). SDM is, in some respects, easy to describe – indeed it is 'what it sounds like', that is, professionals and patients making decisions together. It describes a middle way between a scenario in which the professional makes a clinical decision wholly by themselves with the patient having a completely passive role, and one in which all the decision making is in the hands of the patient and the professional is just a mere ('unthinking') service provider. There may be some exceptional cases where one or other of these scenarios might apply but, for the most part, they are both unacceptable. The former fails to recognise the position of, and to respect, the patient and the latter fails to recognise the position of, and respect, the professional.

In this broad sense of a somehow balanced 'middle way' it is very difficult to object to SDM and it seems to be rightly suited to being treated as a policy imperative. There are so many potential advantages of drawing patient agency more fully into decision-making processes. It is worth first saying a little more about SDM in order to illustrate one policy interpretation of patient choice and some of its advantages.

Of course there are very few scenarios in which patients do not participate in some sense, even in the most paternalistic models of provision. Except where the patient is unconscious they will typically play a role in describing their symptoms and experiences, relating their own health concerns and in providing important data about their clinical history, life circumstances and so on. But other 'layers' of participation are possible. In particular, patients can (a) feed into decision making by sharing their own views and preferences about what they value in life, in relation to the risks and benefits of treatments and in relation to what they would and would not like as outcomes;

(b) participate directly in deliberations and decisions about which lines of treatment (or investigation or referral) might and will be pursued. The advocates of SDM are normally using it to include both these things, but especially (b), and to encourage professionals to be ready to cross the line between (a) and (b). That is, SDM is used to denote something more than 'passive involvement', where the patient is treated as a source of important data; it requires some level of inclusion in the decision-making processes.

There is not one agreed definition of SDM in the literature but the most widely cited accounts describe a process in which professionals and patients work together, both parties share information – the professional contributes their knowledge base, including the evidence about the risks and benefits of treatment options (including no treatment), the patient contributes their account of what matters to them, including their perceptions of various options – and the two parties jointly deliberate about what should happen and try to come to a shared decision (Charles et al, 1997). One formulation of this broad approach has been pithily summarised by some authors as 'evidence-based patient choice' (EBPC) (Edwards and Elwyn, 2009).

There are many things in favour of this approach. In addition to treating patients with respect (which some will say is already sufficient justification), engaging patients in clinical decisions has potential to build their understanding of their conditions and treatments. Also it serves – especially over time in the case of long-term conditions – to build up their motivation and sense of 'ownership', which, as discussed in the last chapter, is also liable to improve levels of adherence (or produce what has been called 'informed adherence') (Horne et al, 2005). More generally, practising this level of participation seems likely to contribute to all of the other ways that people might participate in healthcare. In this context terms like 'empowerment' or 'activation' are sometimes used to indicate the scope for liberating patients from a passive role and mobilising them to use their relevant knowledge and skills – processes that have substantial implications beyond the moment of clinical consultation, for example, for self-management, peer support or service redesign. In addition, the philosophy of 'working together' – or partnership or collaboration – can arguably help to deepen and enhance the quality of professional–patient relationships.

As well as having these benefits for individual patients and healthcare relationships, EBPC has been presented as addressing one of the major macro policy challenges, introduced in the previous chapter, that is, the problem of unwarranted practice variation. How can we even know what treatments are 'needed' or are more 'effective' unless we know what patients actually value, and want to happen, when faced with the evidence about treatments? Indeed Jack Wennberg, the scholar most responsible for identifying practice variation, has cited evidence-informed patient choice as the crucial policy reform needed in health systems:

> Reducing unwarranted variation in preference-sensitive care and establishing the 'right rate' for discretionary surgery and other preference-sensitive interventions require fundamental changes in the doctor–patient relationship and the standards governing the determination of medical necessity: delegated decision-making should be replaced by shared decision-making; and the doctrine of informed patient consent superseded by informed patient choice.
>
> The challenge to policy makers is to promote the transition from delegated decision-making to informed patient choice: to support improvements in clinical science to assure evidence-based patient choice; and encourage practicing physicians and their patients to adopt shared decision-making ... (Foreword to Edwards and Elwyn, 2009)

The reason why shared decision making is often treated as a critically important development, and not just a fad or fashion, is evident in this quote. It can be seen as the confluence and culmination of two independently important currents in the evolution of healthcare – evidence-based medicine (EBM) and respect for patient autonomy (RPA). Both these currents have already had considerable success and achieved the status of mainstream norms. It is now normal for clinicians to be asked to account for their judgements by reference to the best available evidence, and for clinical interventions to proceed only with the voluntary and informed consent of patients. What Wennberg, and others, are pointing out is that neither of these currents can be coherently developed or completed except in conjunction with the other one. In short, EBM depends upon RPA and vice versa. This is because (a) if EBM is about identifying the 'best means to the best outcome', then what counts as 'best', in relation to both means and outcomes, will often actually depend upon patients' values and preferences and these will therefore require elicitation (assuming, for now, that this idea is unproblematic); (b) if we want to be reasonably confident that patients are making a meaningful choice to follow a particular line of treatment, then we need to ensure that they have an understanding of what the processes and outcomes of this course of action, and alternative viable courses, might include, and this depends upon collating and sharing evidence from past experiences with other patients. SDM is thus arguably the logical and optimum way to advance both these agendas.

SDM represents a challenge to, or at least a development of, traditional models of health professionalism and can be regarded as one version of 'new professionalism' (Cribb and Gewirtz, 2015). These new varieties of professional practice highlight the fact that there is no single or fixed 'logic' of professionalism – professionalism is evolving as part of broader social and philosophical transitions. Nonetheless, forms of collaborative working such as SDM can still be broadly consistent with the logic of professionalism in Freidson's sense (introduced in the previous chapter), as a mode of social coordination, in so far as this is contrasted with market or bureaucratic logics. Indeed it could be argued that the animating spirit of SDM is merely a fuller expression or realisation of professionalism in this sense.

Sharing decisions: obstacles, complications and dilemmas

There is still a very significant gap between theory and practice when it comes to SDM. Although there are many examples of healthcare settings where something like SDM is employed and although the broad principles of SDM are widely endorsed, large areas of healthcare practice 'fall short' of SDM. Given the very strong rationale for SDM – which I wish to underline and not to dismiss – it is worth spending some time asking why this is the case. Exploring the reasons behind this theory–practice gap will help to open up the limitations and challenges of 'choice' as the answer to sub-optimal healthcare.

I will briefly describe three of the different kinds of reasons here – first, problems of implementing change; second, problems of scope and specification; and third, problems of evaluation. These different kinds of reasons work in combination but I will separate them out for presentational purposes.

1. Changing practice is often very hard to do. It means confronting the problem of 'path dependency' – the phenomenon that practices tend to carry on along the same tracks despite the introduction of new thinking or new official policy discourses. This is because, as alluded to in earlier chapters, ideas are only one ingredient of practice and depend for their realisation on becoming embodied in socio-material structures (institutional and physical resources, regimes,

equipment, texts, norms and habits and so on). It is comparatively easy to 'rethink' what should happen in the abstract but it is a very much more time-consuming and demanding process to replace the socio-material structures, and these will inevitably continue steering things in the same (old) direction. (An analogy that is often cited here but, if anything, understates the challenge, is the lag between deciding to change the direction of a supertanker and the time and effort required to turn around something with massive momentum.)

Practice change can be studied and illuminated from many angles – it is of interest to specialists in management, psychology and education and is a key focus for inter-disciplinary fields such as 'implementation science'. For a start, there are resource needs and constraints – change requires investment. This includes the time needed for people to consider and adjust to the proposed changes but will often include the availability of resources and tools to facilitate or underpin new forms of practice. In addition there are, as just noted, the established structural, attitudinal and behavioural norms that tend to reinforce current practice and inhibit change, even with an 'in principle' willingness to change. Those who have an interest in health promotion or theories of 'behaviour change' have accumulated very extensive evidence of how difficult it can be for people to make health-related life-style adjustments. Routines and habits are often set fairly solid and people will typically keep travelling along the same grooves unless something substantial occurs to change their environment. Analogous difficulties attach to attempts to change professional–patient relationships. Both professionals and patients have expectations of themselves and of one another. It is no mean feat to overturn these. In other words, the theory–practice gap could be explained by saying that the practical obstacles are simply too substantial to overcome.

2. Equally important forms of inertia or resistance spring from inherent uncertainties about what exactly is required or entailed by the shift to greater patient choice. It is certainly not merely that professionals and patients are resistant to change. And that is not the only source of potential discomfort. It is that they are also unsure about exactly which kinds of change are needed (or – see next section – desirable). These uncertainties link in with much broader debates about the merits and demerits of choice, for example, debates about whether choice can be unwelcome, whether and when people would necessarily 'choose choice' and about whether choice is sometimes incompatible with good care (see, for example, the discussion of Annemarie Mol's work later in this chapter). The positions we

might adopt in these debates depend very much upon how choice is interpreted and enacted and on the broader social and ideological processes that shape versions of choice.

SDM as evidence-based patient choice necessarily focuses on some sub-set of choices. Doctors are not expected to invite all patients, all of the time, into every possible element of decision making that is entailed by their care. They might for example encourage patients to get involved in deciding whether or not a surgical operation is performed, or even what mode of operation to perform, or whether or not, for example, a general or a local anaesthetic is used. But they will not be expected to debate the small variations in anaesthetic drugs or surgical techniques that might be used. This is neither practicable nor required by the rationale for SDM. The crux of SDM is to help patients to participate in decisions that are of significance to them and where they might have relevant preferences that help to determine what should happen. But once we have noted that some strong parameters are drawn around the scope of SDM, then we are bound to wonder about the way the parameters should be drawn.

Of course, patients cannot, in any case, simply choose anything they want to – the very idea of SDM requires that health-professional systems and judgements help to set the boundaries of choice. An analogy that is difficult to avoid here is that patients might be seen as being in the position of diners in a restaurant who are faced with a (necessarily) restricted menu of options – they might be guided through the options and helped to choose according to their preferences; but someone else is compiling the menu. This need not be seen as a problem – it is often the only sensible and responsible path – but it sometimes can be. Where choice applies within a defined option set and not to the making of the option set it is certainly a restricted form of choice. Whether or not this restriction matters depends, for example, upon whether a well-informed observer might judge that other things ought to be on the menu, or how easy it might be to go 'off menu' if that is something that a patient and professional can agree might be helpful.

As well as restrictions to the kinds of choices that patients might be supported to make, the enactment of SDM entails making discriminations about who is in a position to make choices, and the states or circumstances in which it makes sense to expect people to choose. In addition to relatively clear-cut cases where there is judged to be a lack of mental capacity to participate in SDM there are very many less clear-cut cases where it might be judged unwise to ask or expect people to share decisions, except in a qualified way. People who are making high-stakes decisions about their future health and well-being (and these are, as just noted, very much the kinds of instances for which SDM is considered most relevant and important) are rarely in the situation of diners in a restaurant. Whereas the latter are in a relaxed and largely anxiety-free environment and making short-term choices, the former will frequently be making decisions with long-term implications under stress, may be physically uncomfortable or in pain and will often be experiencing significant, and sometimes substantial, emotional and social disequilibrium. Adjusting to episodes of ill-health, and the existential threats they represent, is often very demanding and disorienting – indeed there is no simple line to be drawn between physical and mental ill-health experiences in this regard. This is definitely not a reason to exclude people from decisions that affect their life. The arguments for the importance of SDM stand. However, it is a reason to think carefully about *how to involve* people in decision -making and *how to support* them in the process, including when it is unrealistic to expect active choice making rather than understanding and agreement from patients. I will return to this contrast between a 'consumer' being helped to choose from a menu and a patient helping to choose their care in the next section.

3. Uncertainties about the correct way to interpret and apply patient-choice policies shade into questions about how we should evaluate their application – where and when, for example, are practical enactments of SDM good or bad? Even while remaining convinced about the broad, in principle, justification for the policy aspiration towards an approach like EBPC one can be concerned about the ways in such an approach might misfire, cause harm to, or otherwise undermine, patients. This gives rise to dilemmas for policy makers and professionals. There will sometimes be competing concerns to balance together – the strong arguments for involving patients in decisions pulling in one direction and uncertainties about how far this is feasible, or the risks of sharing the burden of decision making with patients, pulling in the opposite direction. Given these complexities, professionals who are conscientiously interested in advancing patient well-being and in respecting patient autonomy will not necessarily endorse SDM in a blanket way. Rather, they will want to see how it might be implemented in specific instances and whether these instances actually qualify as both respectful and caring.

In addition most people would accept that professionals sometimes need to circumscribe the range of choices available. Although I am not discussing it here, it is worth stressing this fact. Indeed the whole idea of SDM can put clinicians and patients on a collision course – this can be explained in terms of them operating with different conceptions of health or, more generally, by them simply having different interests and purposes (Owens and Cribb, 2012). Partnership, in short, will sometimes be associated with conflict, rather than harmony – I will discuss this further in Chapter Six. There are various reasons for possible tensions between professional and patient agendas. Professionals have a role in, and are accountable for, protecting patients' interests and safeguarding public health (which means ruling out choices that are damaging to individual or population health) – that is the very core of their professionalism. And in any health system or institution that has an element of 'cost sharing'[1] professionals, along with system administrators, have a duty to avoid unjustified expenditure and to reduce the number of wasteful choices. Both of these factors come to a head in situations where individuals might choose interventions with resource implications that professionals judge to be unnecessary and risky. An example which affects many people's lives and which gets media attention from time to time is the advice on caesarean sections – in the UK the advice from the National Institute for Health and Care Excellence (last updated in 2011) is that caesareans can be provided for women who choose them even if they are not medically necessary. By contrast, the World Health Organization guidance recommends that caesareans need to be medically necessary because the operation 'can cause significant complications, disability or death' and divert resources away from areas where they may be more needed. (*The Times*, 11 April 2015). Different policy makers and professionals may come to different decisions about the best way to regulate and achieve balance in these cases, but what they simply cannot do is abnegate responsibility for attending to these dilemmas.

These considerations help to give a concrete sense to the notion of the 'common good', introduced in the previous chapter. Albeit this is a compound and contested notion we can see how it might sometimes be understood by reference to something like the protection of public health (which collectively benefits everyone). More generally, it might be understood as pointing to an 'overall good' – albeit interpreted through a number of competing lenses – such as something like an 'aggregate good', or a fair distribution of benefits and burdens. In other words, these considerations remind us that individual choice cannot be straightforwardly defended in unqualified ways but is better seen as something that should be circumscribed by (or perhaps should itself be understood as one element of) the 'common good'.

The idea that acts of individual choice need not be seen in isolation is, of course, built into the language of SDM. Professionals, for the reasons discussed above, often have a role in mediating the way decisions are experienced by patients and sometimes in supporting them in decision making, or at least ensuring that appropriate forms of support are available when needed. That is to say, it is not just the consequences of choice making that are social; the process of choice making can be seen as a social one. Given the importance that can be attached to the supportive function of professionals and others, as well as the need to apply any choice policies flexibly and responsively, some might prefer to avoid using the word 'choice' here altogether and talk rather about participation or partnership in decision making.

The language of SDM thus has the potential to stretch much further than an emphasis on patient choice – especially where this is understood simply as the wholly independent 'picking from a menu' notion. There are broader and richer conceptions of SDM that stress the 'shared' elements of choice making, the mutuality and collaborative processes – whether involving family, friends or professionals – that can help to provide a platform for patient autonomy (Cribb and Entwistle, 2011). It is a commonplace of our day-to-day existence that our so-called 'personal' autonomy is socially underpinned. We do not generally reason about things, manage or draw upon our emotions, or practically make decisions in isolation; rather, we do so by thinking, feeling, working and being alongside others. A number of theorists, including most prominently feminist theorists, have sought to emphasise this relational dimension of autonomy and have coined the language of 'relational autonomy' as a way to capture this phenomenon (Mackenzie and Stoljar, 2000). The key insight here is that the agency and autonomy of individuals do not arise out of nothing but are developed and enjoyed as social accomplishments. The possibilities of, and scope for, individual action are products of people's socio-material opportunities. This includes the fact that individuals typically act as one of a nexus of agents; a nexus that simultaneously both enables and constrains personal autonomy. This means, for example, that it is simply a mistake to assume that individuals who are 'left alone' to choose are exercising more autonomy than those who make decisions in concert with others. But it also makes it clear that – while personal autonomy can be meaningfully supported by professionals, families or others – there are dangers in assuming that all practices that look like 'support' enhance autonomy, because they can carry risks of powerfully placed actors actually inhibiting the capacity and confidence of individuals.

Broader controversies about choice

The uncertainties rehearsed above connect to a set of broader controversies about choice. In turn these are entangled with debates about our vision of the healthcare system and of the wider society we want to live in. A heavy emphasis on patients choosing their own treatments may, for example, be regarded with scepticism by those who are worried about the effect of liberal individualist norms – sometimes including the assumption or active promotion of a pervasive 'consumerism' – on our framing of health policy. Why, that is, should we be thinking about allocating healthcare goods as if the health system was nothing more than a collection of separate individual choosers? If we are interested in health as a social good, or a common good, might it not be better, for example, to place more emphasis on the ways in which groups of patients might work in a solidaristic spirit to help to co-design service provision, or even help to recreate a new vision, and participate in new practices, for healthcare? There is, as many would stress, a difference between policies being framed around the idea of patients as individual consumers and them being framed around the idea of patients as citizens. It is perfectly fair to argue that both things should be possible and that they are not necessarily incompatible with one another. However there are many potential tensions between individual and collective participation in health services and it is necessary to look closely at what is included and stressed (or excluded and marginalised) in policy proposals to judge where the balance of emphasis lies. And, as with SDM, determining the right balance depends both on issues of general principle and on the realities of enactment.

The scope for debate and disagreement can be seen even in instances where individual consumer choice is universally accepted as a relevant principle. Even in the archetypical case of a restaurant menu it is not uncommon for people to complain about the size or complexity of the menu ('There is too much choice!') or to find ways of simplifying or evading the choice ('What do you suggest?' 'I'll have what you have'). The psychologist Barry Schwartz (2004) has charted the ways in which the broader marketplace for commodities can be experienced as a disbenefit to people. Schwartz is not himself questioning the claim that market choice is a net contributor to human well-being but, rather, addressing the psychological 'costs' of choice that arise at least in relation to some choice-making situations. These situations may occur, for example, where there is an extensive range of choice, where considerable time and effort is required to differentiate between options and where the taxing and somewhat indeterminate process of selection effectively leaves the chooser with the dissatisfied feeling that they have probably made the wrong choice!

Of course there are also more social, ethical and political critiques of the way some goods are commodified and marketised, which lead to more reflective and critical forms of dissatisfaction. For example, someone might point to the fact that their local convenience store has lots of 'choice' of heavily processed foods, including dozens of kinds of potato chips, but no fresh fruit and vegetables – the choices some wish to make are not available to them and the choices they are offered are not ones they want or, they could reasonably argue, need. Such critics are likely to argue, more generally, that although choice is legitimated as being oriented towards and benefiting the choosers we always need to ask whose interests the production of choice serves. These ideological critiques overlap with sociological readings that question the norm of individual self-determination and 'self-making' through choice, referred to in Chapter One, as a feature of advanced liberal societies. In particular there are long-standing and influential sociological critiques of the 'dark side' of discourses of individual 'self-making' in welfare policy and practice. These discourses that underpin and legitimate policies of participation and partnership are seen more sceptically from, for example, neo-Marxist and Foucauldian sociological perspectives. Neo-Marxist readings highlight the dangers of superficially benign norms amounting to 'victim-blaming' and, more broadly, reproducing forms of inequality and oppression (Navarro, 2009), whereas Foucauldian readings famously highlight and interrogate the way such discourses deploy individual autonomy and the 'responsibilisation' of individuals as a form of 'governance': promoting autonomy but simultaneously, as Rose puts it, 'enwrapping these autonomised actors within new forms of control' (Rose, 1989). These perspectives thus help to provide some theoretical articulation to concerns about choice – that devolving responsibility to individuals through the language of autonomy can be illusory (for example, because they are thereby given identities as 'choosers' that restrict and burden them), can amount to the unwarranted 'off-loading' of responsibility and (especially where individuals are unsupported or otherwise disadvantaged) may simply further reproduce health inequalities.

Concerns about the limitations of, and problems associated with, choice are exacerbated in the contexts of healthcare, where the idea that health is a commodity that patients consume is very widely questioned. Many people challenge the appropriateness of a market or consumerist model to situations where the individual consumers are often vulnerable and where there are substantial differentials of power and knowledge between consumers and providers. The worry is that markets do not serve the interests of vulnerable patients and even that market structures and climates have a tendency to 'crowd out' other values – for example, those relating to trust, protection and support – that are, in this instance, essential to looking after the interests of patients (Sandel, 2012). Furthermore, to the extent that clinical decision making was entirely equated with individual consumer choice on a market model, then the very idea of health professionalism as an independent safeguard would be lost. The evolving logic(s) of professionalism can be both inflected and sustained by collaborative models of working, but professionalism would be dissolved altogether if SDM was collapsed into pure consumerism.

On the other hand, some policy makers in non-market systems have sought to use market mechanisms, with the avowed intent of challenging the relative power and vested interests of healthcare providers. For example, a programme of market-inspired reforms, running since 1991 in England, have sought to create 'quasi-markets' within the overall NHS system by encouraging and enabling greater choice of, and competition between, providers (Le Grand, 2007). Some of these reforms relate to matters of convenience – such as more flexibility about time and place of appointments – which are significant from a 'consumer satisfaction' perspective but have little effect on the substantive questions about the nature of healthcare provided. People making choices around the convenience of accessing services, given their personal circumstances and schedules, are not obviously in a very different position from people choosing any kind of service for its convenience. It is obvious why some people would think a consumer-research model might work well here. (Although it is worth noting that not everyone has the same resources or interest in being a demanding consumer and that the consumer model may suit, and benefit, some much more than others.) Other kinds of choices relate to more substantive goods. For example, there have been attempts within the same health system to give patients more choice over which institutions they are referred to, informed by access to various kinds of performance data about possible providers (at least in principle, although the practice has been very slow and patchy).

These contrasting examples suggest that whether or not the use of choice strategies can be defended and made to work might depend very much on the kinds of choices in question. Choice of appointment times is an instance where it seems feasible and desirable to 'mobilise' patients to encourage institutions to be more flexible and responsive. Choice of professionals on the basis of performance data is much more contentious – how far is it wise and feasible to attempt to 'flatten' the knowledge and power hierarchy and to wholly replace professional referral with patient choice in this case, and in particular how far is it credible to do so on the basis of necessarily simplified 'user friendly' performance data (which raises doubts about its validity or robustness)? Here it seems that there is some evidence that patients do value choice, but, at the same time, they value it less than the general protection of quality across the system. Fotaki (2014), for example, argues that 'The evidence also shows that as citizens and users of the NHS patients are more concerned about retaining the public and universal aspects of their health system than having a choice over the providers of their care.' Once again this might seem to be an area where the availability of individual support or collective support as a common good might often be more valued by patients than 'isolated' choice.

The brief cases with which I began the chapter also illustrate these contrasts. Ella and Grant are effectively 'shopping around' for a service that suits their life-style and availability. Here the analogy with other kinds of consumer choices seems broadly apt; although, as just noted, we should be mindful that these kinds of active choices will be easier for, and more 'second nature' to, some than others. Stefan, by contrast, is facing a substantive decision about his health and is being encouraged to help make a choice about the urgency of a referral. The implication is that the doctor thinks it will make comparatively little difference if the referral is postponed a little and provides a chance for Stefan to say if he is feeling too anxious to wait. This is broadly analogous to the caesarean example above, where there may be some tension between two vantage points. In Stefan's case the doctor does not think the quick referral is strictly necessary but there is enough uncertainty about the matter for him or her to see Stefan's feelings and preferences – because they reflect what matters to Stefan – as relevant to making a good decision. Anya and her family are in a very different situation. They face an extremely difficult decision – they are the ones who will have to go down whatever fear-laden path is taken and it is crucial that they understand the alternative paths and contribute to the directions chosen. Unfortunately, however, the 'choices' are far from easy. Indeed they coincide with what I described in the last chapter as the central normative tension in the philosophical transition – what counts as too much medicine? Anya is worn out and overwhelmed. Her experience most probably feels nothing at all like 'shopping around' for solutions.

Providing choice is not caring

In a wonderfully insightful book that draws on ethnographic fieldwork and the author's own experiences and reflections Annemarie Mol (2008) has encouraged us to be sceptical about the widespread policy support for patient choice. Mol is not attempting to legislate for all situations and for all facets of patient choice but is, rather, using case studies of people being treated for and living with diabetes to illuminate the inadequacy of the idea of choice in specific cases and settings. However, her overall thesis has general relevance and importance. Specifically, her analysis shows that there is a severe limit to how complete an account of the processes and experiences of healthcare can be presented in the language of choice. It is not, she argues, that talk of choice lacks any relevance but, rather, that it fails to capture very much of what is most important about good care. In addition, as noted in the discussion above, there is something about the nature of care that means that approaching caring situations and relationships through the frame of choice risks being a positively uncaring thing to do.

Mol's critical analysis is applied to both to consumerist and citizenship conceptions of choice. The differences between these conceptions are important but they both reflect sets of assumptions that, Mol argues, do not 'fit' the sets of experiences and practices she is writing about. If we actually pay attention to caring practices, then we can see that they express, and are underpinned by, a different rationale or 'logic' than the rationale embodied in dominant framings of choice. The 'logic of choice', according to Mol, while superficially plausible, actually imports unhelpful norms and expectations from other arenas into the arena of healthcare. The essential issue for people struggling with ill-health, often living with damaged bodies and damaged identities and facing uncertain futures, is not that they are 'given choices' but that they are not neglected. It is neither reasonable nor kind to expect people facing such turbulence to navigate their way through a series of alternative 'pathways' independently. The practices of care that overcome neglect must certainly respect and work with the agency of patients, but the expressions of agency need not, and arguably should not in general, take the same form as the kinds of choice making expected from consumers or citizens.

There are many reasons for, or ways of understanding, the divergences here. It is not just that it is sometimes uncaring to treat patients as independent choosers but also that there are very often no clearly defined 'pathways' to pick from. Caring is an 'art' that depends upon being responsive to emerging and unstable needs, continuing trial and adaptation as circumstances and experiences change, and collectively 'piecing together' provisional adjustments and forms of support. There may well be some 'big choices' but (a) these occur in the midst of an indefinitely large number of decisions – involving various health professionals, family and other carers and the patient in an ongoing process of collective choreography – and (b) even these big choices do not need to be 'handed over' to the patient acting as if they were an isolated decision-making unit. In so far as individual choice making is called for within healthcare, then, it should be provided in a context where patients are offered consolation, kindness and encouragement and are helped to identify, and come to terms with, who they are and what they think. Finding one's way through treatment and day-to-day living with ill-health is not a matter of plugging one's pre-existing preferences into the menu or decision tree provided. There is often no menu but only a series of improvisations, and one's own preferences often have to emerge, take shape, be moulded and remoulded rather than simply uncovered as if they were pre-existing 'facts'.

Thus, by closely attending to the purposes of, and the complex nature of, caring practices – the avoidance of neglect, the uncertain destinations and routes, the multiple and joint forms of agency entailed – Mol shows the dangers of placing too much emphasis on certain models of choice. Her account does not deny the central importance of patient autonomy or patient responsibility but it warns us against simply analysing this importance in individualist terms or as about the transfer of the locus of control from one place to another. Rather than trying to remake healthcare by unquestioningly borrowing a rationale and set of practices from elsewhere, Mol asks whether we should not first understand the nature of care and the kinds of practices it requires. Once we have done so, then perhaps we should tentatively ask, as Mol goes on to do later in her book, whether some of the lessons of reflecting on the 'logic of care' might not helpfully inform practices in other arenas, and also help to frame the design of healthcare institutions and climates:

> if I argue that healthcare deserves to be improved on its own terms, this does not mean that these terms only makes sense inside healthcare. They might (be made to) move around..... More generally, one may wonder what kinds of institutional conditions are needed for care to flourish. (Mol, 2008, p 92)

Mol's analysis does not contradict the value of a movement like SDM. But it does reinforce concerns about SDM being interpreted and implemented in narrow terms. Her account resonates much more closely with what I discussed earlier as broader and more collaborative interpretations of SDM – in which some choice making is both shared and supported – rather than those interpretations with a sharp division of labour between option providers and option consumers.

More generally this analysis chimes with broader critiques of the presence of liberal, individualist norms in healthcare. These norms can be seen as built into some dominant constructions of biomedicine, especially those produced and propagated by pressures towards marketised or consumerist versions of health services. What are needed are different ways of thinking and talking. The clues to these alternatives are around if we look for them – in the diffuse but vital practices of caring and humanity often manifest in the work of health professionals, and rooted even more broadly in the everyday practices of kindness, compassion and support within families and communities. These alternatives do not consist in offering 'no choice' but set choice making in context.

Patient agency – correcting, reinforcing or revising biomedicine?

The various policy and social movements that seek to find ways of harnessing the agency of patients and carers are of great importance. More specifically, the moral and practical importance of supporting and respecting patient autonomy can no longer be in doubt. However – as with all healthcare goods – what matters is not only the abstract good but the ways in which the good is interpreted and translated into practice. It is worth distinguishing between two different emphases in the broad shift from professional paternalism to patient autonomy. One emphasis is on the transfer of decision-making authority and responsibility from the individual of the professional to the individual of the patient. A contrasting emphasis is on a shift away from a picture of separate individual agents to notions of richer relationships, including more focus upon collaborative or partnership working. I would suggest that there is a place for both these emphases but that great care is needed to achieve the right balances between them in the right contexts and cases. Personal autonomy is properly established as a key value in healthcare but it does not always help to think of this as a kind of individual sovereignty; rather, there is much wisdom in the recognition of the relational dimension of autonomy.

What I have been arguing here, and illustrating through the case of patient choice, is that some of the powerful ideas and norms that shape healthcare (such as in this case expert authority and paternalism) do need 'correcting' or 'balancing' with other ideas, but that in the process we need to be careful not to generate too many other problems and imbalances. The historically dominant forms of biomedically oriented healthcare need some moderating by more person-centred conceptions of healthcare; and one element of this moderation should undoubtedly be a greater emphasis on patient autonomy, involvement and collaborative working. Within this mix there is a place for patient choice. But we must not treat the idea of 'choice' as a solution except in a highly qualified way. And unless we proceed wisely and cautiously, the norms embedded in influential examples and approaches to the provision of choice, including some forms of SDM, will do their own damage to healthcare. Choice may be part of the answer to a 'cure imperative', but a 'choice imperative' is potentially just as hostile to the nature of good care.

Indeed the very idea that choice is a corrective to the biomedical model needs to be problematised. Some of the best arguments for the importance of patient choice – such as those rehearsed above about 'evidence-based patient choice' (EBPC) – might be understood as about the reinforcement of a biomedical model. As noted earlier, a scientific approach to collecting data and undertaking the optimum technical and practical reasoning to define the best-available clinical intervention and outcome is inherently incomplete without knowledge of patient preferences. Without an active component of eliciting patient values and preferences, then, biomedical reasoning will fall short: it can reasonably aim to make valid judgements about people's bodies and what might happen to them, but it cannot make valid claims about the course of people's lives and what should be done.

The greater incorporation of patient values and preferences into the biomedical model can be seen in both a positive and a negative light. The positive readings have been discussed already, and they are fundamentally important. They are about increasing the chance of individuals getting the treatments and outcomes they value and not the ones they don't value. And the implementation of SDM also increases the potential and power of medicine to improve health services for the whole population and not just for specific individuals (Mulley et al, 2012a). This is because, if and when patients' informed preferences are elicited routinely, it becomes possible to use these aggregated preferences to revise service plans and offers more systematically. If 90% of the relevant population prefers operation x over operation y, then macro- and meso-level adjustments can be made to the allocation of resources and institutional efforts. Furthermore, this provides a useful information base for individuals on similar illness trajectories. The broad findings about preferences among the relevant sub-populations, and the reasons lying behind them, can be (carefully) shared with individuals facing similar choices *as part of* the support that is offered them in their deliberation.

But these same processes of 'harnessing' patient preferences can be seen in a negative light; at least this is the case if SDM is interpreted in a narrow sense. In particular they can be interpreted as reproducing some of more instrumentalist and technicist currents in biomedicine. From this vantage point the forms of patient inclusion or involvement embodied in narrow forms of SDM are very limited. They basically involve the incorporation of patients into scientific medicine and associated forms of medical reasoning and practice rather than the full 'meeting' of medical and patient perspectives and agendas. The argument would be that, at least in some cases, the patient might be seen as being recruited to underpin and strengthen clinical reasoning – as a further 'tool' in the reasoning process – rather than as a genuine partner.

The extent of this kind of concern depends on how SDM is interpreted or enacted in practice. To return to the 'menu' analogy, if the full extent of the contribution from the patient is to be expected to pick from a pre-defined and limited menu of options, then it could be argued that the patient is not so much collaborating in a process but is, rather, 'servicing' a system, albeit one from which they might well be benefiting. We need to look at both the general and specific operationalisation of policy initiatives to evaluate them. In the case of SDM, for example, there are now very many 'decision aids' or other 'decision support tools' available to help operationalise patient involvement in decision making. These are tools designed to help inform and involve patients. They can helpfully summarise the nature of conditions, treatment options, intended outcomes and possible side-effects and can 'translate' complex information, including evidence relating to risks and probabilities, into a form that is accessible and practical for lay people. These tools can help to turn a policy aspiration into a practical reality. Nonetheless this is a demanding task. Such tools need developing for, or adapting to, diverse settings, illness trajectories and people. They need to be embedded in working contexts, and this includes familiarising staff with, or training staff in, their use, including their strengths and limitations, and reviewing and updating practices from time to time. Not least, the effectiveness of such tools will often depend upon how they are used, and how skilfully they are mediated or interpreted by professionals.

The dangers of poor usage or mediation are very real. The tools themselves, unless we subject them to critical scrutiny, may be out of date or contain misleading emphases or unintended 'steers' (perhaps for some audiences more than others). In addition, the use of the tools generates its own hazards and needs careful monitoring and evaluation. If decision aids, or other such tools, are used to help underpin and contribute to more open-ended and responsive professional–patient exchanges, then they can play an invaluable role. If they are used to replace or displace that open-endedness they may do as much harm as good. The move towards higher levels of collaborative working between professionals and patients, if it is to be truly meaningful, should not just smooth the processes of, or provide data for, clinical reasoning but should enhance the breadth and depth of communication between parties.

The shortcoming could be expressed like this: in many instances of SDM some steps have been taken to 'involve' the patient in the world, concerns and projects of the health professional, but limited or no steps have been taken to involve the professional in the world, concerns and projects of the patient (Donetto and Cribb, 2011). This latter involves 'extending' the perspectives and sensibilities of biomedical actors. Such broader forms of collaborative relationships and working embody some degree of open-endedness and they potentially extend well beyond SDM. Health professionals will potentially have to engage with the perspectives, uncertainties, hopes and fears of patients and need to take seriously those trajectories and problems that derive from the lives and projects of their patients and not solely from clinical agendas. This reorientation of the idea of collaboration or joint working – with more emphasis on professionals participating in the activities and contexts of patients rather than the other way around – is a much more significant revision to the conventional biomedical model. In this context the role and status of professionals will be more fluid. They will have to be ready to see themselves in a range of different ways; for example, not just as experts or facilitators but also as learners from, and co-citizens with, the publics they serve. This degree of reorientation and fluidity is considerable, but it is arguably critical to the success of healthcare following the health, social and philosophical transitions discussed earlier.

As we broaden our attention away from treatment decision making and consider the whole of the experience and management of illness in an era where long-term conditions are a major factor, then the perspectives and agency of patients and publics can no longer be seen as an important 'add on' but become the crux of the matter. This is, for example, what lies behind the recognition of 'support for self-management' as a critically important current in health policy. Like SDM, this is a policy area where the centrality of the agency of service users has come to be widely understood and embraced (Entwistle and Cribb, 2013). In this case the telling language of 'self-management' or 'self-care' stems from an acknowledgement not only that people are, by necessity, left to 'manage' most of the time without direct system input, but also that there is often much that individuals and families can do to enhance their experiences and lives that both complements and transcends what can be achieved by healthcare professionals and institutions. But if professionals are going to effectively support self-management, then they will need to find ways – albeit within some (evolving) conception of their own professionalism – of orienting their own agendas and efforts to the agendas and efforts of patients. Unless this happens there is a real risk of more restricted (for example, narrowly biomedical or target driven) professional agendas being imposed on patients (sometimes with damaging consequences) in the name of support (Morgan et al, 2017). This degree of responsiveness and accommodation may seem a very ambitious, or perhaps even unrealistic, vision of the role of health professionals but it is not an empty vision. Indeed it is one that follows from a conception of healthcare that encompasses 'care' and not just 'health outputs' narrowly understood.

Conclusion

Hopefully, one of the insights that have been reinforced by this chapter is that there is no easy way to make healthcare 'person-centred'. Even if we take an interpretation of person-centredness that focuses largely on agency, rather than on other aspects of persons, then this should not be equated with patient choice in a narrow sense. Agency can refer to various forms of collective agency, and 'choices' are not necessarily focused on specific treatment decisions but can relate to the shaping of policies and the providing of services and care. Furthermore, as we have seen, even in the restricted case of individual disease management (the main focus of this chapter) there are reasons to be concerned about interpreting agency as choice, given its potentially uncaring effects. Moreover, in considering the challenges of translating choice into practice, including the normative disputes about when choice is a good thing, we are reminded that agency is only one, albeit important, aspect of persons and thus 'responsiveness to agency' is only one dimension of 'responsiveness to persons'. The different dimensions of person-centredness – summarised in the previous chapter as including responsiveness to vulnerability and suffering, the depth and multi-faceted nature of individuals, people's social constitution and relatedness, as well as their agency – need to be considered holistically. Persons are complex wholes and any interpretation of person-centred care that abstracts one element of concern and makes it 'trumps' will fail to do justice to this complexity. In particular, as will be argued more fully in the next chapter, we need to be wary of the 'individualising' and 'transactional' assumptions that run through some interpretations of person-centredness.

Moving away from the reductionism associated with narrow biomedical models is necessary if we want to do justice to persons and what matters to them. But in so doing we enter territory that is both contested and less well charted by health policy. We are only part way in the transition towards a health system that attaches as much weight to the agency of patients and publics as it does to the agency of professionals and system leaders. And the reason for this is not simple slowness or resistance but because we are – wisely – unclear about what would count as a successful destination. It is already clear that notions of both system effectiveness and equity need to evolve. Although it is very important that healthcare interventions 'work' by producing the clinical effects intended, this is no longer sufficient to judge a service effective. What matters in the emerging context is that a service produces results that reflect the values and preferences of the people treated.

In this context there are thus potentially 'extra' forms of inequity that arise where there are differential opportunities to be listened to or to participate; or when some voices but not others are supported or heard. This is but one example of the many areas of uncertainty and debate thrown up by the healthcare transition under discussion – that is, how should competing conceptions of both effectiveness and equity be weighed in the balance? These debates cannot be resolved by purely empirical or technical methods because they rest upon normative and philosophical questions. I have sketched out some of these questions in this chapter. How far should disaggregated individual values determine what should be done, rather than some more collective conception of what matters? If we want to provide services that best 'fit' individuals, then how far is eliciting their preferences a good and practicable guide to doing so? I will investigate the relevance of these and related questions further in the next two chapters as I continue to explore the potential implications of the transition towards person-centred care.

Note

[1]   Not just 'single payer' systems but often in insurance-based or managed-care systems.

FOUR

Systems and lives

In this chapter I will be exploring some of the things that are entailed by calls for anti-reductionism or 'holism' in health policy. In particular I will be considering what is sometimes called the 'social context' of health. Many reforming currents in health policy are informed by, and draw attention to, the importance of seeing health – including clinical medicine and individual well-being – in social terms. It has, for example, become a truism in health services quality-improvement work that a realistic prospect of change depends upon 'systems thinking' – analysing and addressing the broad range of factors that shape the practices we are hoping to improve. We can see this in relation to reforming ideas such as shared decision-making and support for self-management, discussed in the last chapter. Implementing such reforms depends upon paying attention to, and often reworking, the habits and expectations of both professionals and patients and these, in turn, are shaped by institutional (and broader social) norms and cultures and by material factors such as the design of physical spaces and the availability of supportive resources.

Systems thinking has strong resonances and overlaps with traditions in public health and health promotion which also, of course, look at health in social terms, including as something that needs addressing at a population level. Specifically, expertise used in designing and implementing clinically based public health services such as vaccination and screening is also relevant to attempts to strengthen other clinical services: for example, those relating to the management of long-term conditions, that depend upon such things as the reliable use of demographic data; effective but sensitive communication with patients (such as being called and re-called for appointments); and consistent monitoring and evaluation of results. More broadly, insights from public health and health-promotion perspectives have come to be seen as of fundamental relevance to reorienting health policy. This is because it is now widely understood that people's length and quality of life – including their risks of, experiences of, access to treatment for and capacity to 'manage' diseases and ill-health – is substantially determined by the social conditions of their lives and requires us to think about broader health ecologies, including the inequalities they give rise to, and not just formal health systems. Health inequalities take a variety of shapes and forms but any attempts, however modest, to address them require a focus on the social context of health and well-being.

Lying behind these crucial types of insight is, arguably, an even more general awareness of the way each of our lives – our values, our identities, our biographies, our economic and cultural resources and the way we make sense of and 'own' these things – is shaped by the social worlds that make us who we are. When two people come face to face in a consultation or a care setting there is a danger that we focus only on immediate and surface personal characteristics and interpersonal transactions. This misses out on a great deal – the long and compound social trajectories (that extend far beyond the transitory clinical encounters) that shape people and their interactions and the multi-faceted ways that they can relate to, or fail to relate to, one another. These richer social realities need acknowledgement in discussions about reform.

At the end of the chapter I will return to systems thinking – and its connection to conceptions of effectiveness and efficiency. But before that I will discuss health promotion and the organisation of clinical care in order to investigate some of the implications of the anti-reductionist currents in person-centred models – the insistence that persons are (both 'outwardly' and 'inwardly') socially constituted. If we are to move beyond, or at least complement, the reductionism embodied in the heavy emphasis upon clinical disease management within healthcare, then we need to apply different, and more wide-angled, lenses. For a start this means thinking about physical and mental health and well-being at the same time, and understanding the many interconnections between the different facets of well-being (Royal College of Psychiatrists, 2010). In so doing we need to be ready, as summarised above, to think about systems and ecologies. This includes thinking about populations and communities, and it also involves thinking about persons as relational or social beings. The underlying story of the chapter will have strong echoes of the previous one while following a rather different path. In short, I want to underline the general value of holism as a reforming idea while, at the same time, highlighting the complications and contests that it opens up for would-be reformers. This is essentially the same argument I wanted to make about the turn to patient autonomy (which indeed might itself be understood as an element of holism) for policy solutions. What I have roughly summarised as aspirations towards more person-centred care are motivated by a number of key ideas. Each of these ideas is valuable and helps to point in the direction of better healthcare; but none of these ideas is itself unproblematic. Rather, each produces new challenges and dilemmas.

Whole systems or whole persons? The threats of depersonalisation and exclusion

The central complication facing anyone who wishes to rethink the orientation of healthcare, and the balance of provision, along more holistic lines is that 'holism' is open to a variety of interpretations. Indeed, for the most part, holism is deliberately advocated in self-consciously open-ended ways and by way of contrast with what it is not (that is, as moving beyond reductionism), rather than in a programmatic and carefully specified way. Even where the idea is specified there is still considerable scope for differences in emphasis. This applies, for example, to those who draw upon or apply the 'biopsychosocial model' of health (Engel, 1977). For instance, the thoughtful and relatively systematised model of holistic healthcare offered by Derek Wade (Wade, 2009), which applies a biopsychosocial model, sees the person as made up of the interactions between bodily organs, the body as a whole, the physical environment and the social environment and argues that personal health and illness itself needs to be studied and addressed against four sets of contextual factors – specifically personal, physical, social and temporal contexts. This kind of framework highlights the breadth of relevant and interconnecting factors but certainly allows for a range of interpretive possibilities and emphases.

A very important area of tension contained within the move towards holism – and one that I will come back to throughout this chapter – is the way in which 'the personal' and 'the social' may sometimes seem to pull in different directions. This connects with the realisation, mentioned in the last chapter, that we can stress either the 'separability' or 'inseparability' of persons – treat people as distinct from one another or as co-constitutive of one another. Some people might reasonably wonder, for example, whether the use of systems thinking or public health perspectives in the introduction to this chapter are really examples of the kind of holistic thinking needed in healthcare. Surely, they will argue, what matters most in trying to transcend the most limiting instances of a biomedical model is the recovery of the individual personhood of the patient and the professional? From this perspective it seems that a focus on broader social contexts or even immediate social conditions could simply miss the point. Thinking back to the discussion of care in the last chapter, one of the key things highlighted there was the importance of persons 'being attended to' or 'recognised' (or, in Mol's terms, not being 'neglected'), and this being arguably both ethically and practically prior to people's being allocated to, or actively choosing, the correct care pathways. This suggests both that recognising individual personhood is crucial and also that this depends upon certain kinds of interpersonal relationships. I will return to this notion – that our basic existential or ontological relationship to persons needs to be considered in our attempts to escape reductionism – later in the chapter, and particularly in the discussion of Habermas.

One way of approaching the worry that social lenses might produce depersonalisation is through Goffman's (1961) analysis of 'total institutions' (a somewhat extreme, but for that very reason useful, category). This is a concept that Goffman applied to only a restricted set of historically specific cases, such as certain prison and mental hospital regimes, but that has subsequently been applied, by analogy, to a much broader range of healthcare settings (Thomas, 2002). The notion here is that the institutionalisation of care sometimes seems to depend upon a high level of compliance from people who are – in the case of hospitalisation – literally and metaphorically 'stripped' of their social identities, social status and privacy and made subject to the powerful norms and requirements of the institution (albeit in order to help restore them to better functioning). The clear risk is something like the dehumanisation of the people subjected to these processes. Of course even very large contemporary hospitals, let alone other smaller and more community-based healthcare institutions, will normally make efforts not to conform to this strong version of institutionalisation, but the model nonetheless retains some relevance. We retain a sense that 'fitting in' to an institution can mean 'losing' something of ourselves. This applies not only to stereotypical cases like the army but to any clearly regulated settings, which we often describe, whether favourably or disparagingly, in 'army-like' terms. Is there perhaps some fundamental incompatibility between the needs of systems and the needs of persons, or more generally between population agendas and priorities, on the one hand, and those of particular groups or specific individuals, on the other? This rather diffuse question, or perhaps cluster of questions, will animate much of the subsequent discussion in this chapter.

In approaching some of the balances between systems and individual persons the army is not a bad example to start from. First, it is clear that most social institutions are not as hierarchically organised, as strongly regulated or as oriented around common goals as the armed services are. Many institutions – universities are a reasonable example – are, at least on the face of it, organised around some more liberal conception of 'option freedom' and both foster and respond to expressions of personal autonomy. In addition, most social institutions do not make as extensive a set of demands on individuals as the army; for example, even most workplaces operate with a more circumscribed level of role and time commitment (daily or long term), with more scope to 'escape' the demands of the institution. Second, even in the case of the army, there is no clear-cut contradiction between the needs and purposes of the system and those of the persons who make it up. Many people would defend the benefits of the army in supporting the personal development – character qualities, capabilities, broad well-being – of individual soldiers and even in supporting and fostering a capacity for rich and critical kinds of autonomy within shared frameworks of solidarity and purpose.

Indeed it seems that when we look more closely there are many commonalities between apparently diverse social institutions. There are, of course, very great differences of emphases, but institutions depend, by definition, both on harnessing the agency and commitments of people and on some level of coordination and cohesion that both enables, and provides constraints upon, the exercise of that agency. How we evaluate the balances struck between the kinds and quantities of constraints and option freedoms within institutions will partly depend upon the purposes of those institutions but will also depend, more broadly, on our social and political ideologies. Not everyone attaches the same weight to the importance of people's having a very large range of option freedoms and not everyone is equally sceptical about the innate costs of some conformity – this is even more evident if we look cross-culturally at people with diverse social identities.

But this takes us on to another set of concerns about the social consequences of systems and institutions – the differential impacts they may have on different groups of people. In the case of universities, for example, there are well-known patterns of 'institutional discrimination'. These relate to every facet of social inequality – economic, cultural and political (Fraser, 1996; Fraser, 2013); for example, in relation to women or for people with specific minority ethnic identities there are ongoing struggles about: fair distribution of places and opportunities for progression; equal recognition of people's identities, including the reflection of multiple forms of diversity in curricula; and equal representation in the membership and activities of the political groupings that make decisions about distribution and recognition (including decisions about who makes the decisions). As is now well understood this can, but does not need to, be seen a product of deliberate or self-conscious sexism or racism. The norms and expectations built into social institutions (within the army and education or health systems) – and the collective and individual habits of people within them – are built up around assumptions that continually reinforce advantage. The fact that many of these forms of discrimination are indirect does not make their consequences any less malign or any less palpable to those who suffer from them, nor does it absolve role-holders within institutions from collective responsibility for addressing them.

The patterns of relative inclusion/exclusion created by institutions are complex. Most obviously, institutions will often end up reinforcing recognised social inequalities such as those relating to gender, 'race', class, disability or sexual orientation – while, at the same time, perhaps genuinely attempting to challenge or ameliorate them. But there are very many more subtle ways in which institutions can be relatively blind to the variations between groups of people (whether or not relating to these broad categories of identity difference) and can thereby risk reinforcing or creating social inequalities. For example, differences in people's readiness to engage in certain styles of communication (for example, confident performances of argument and debate in universities; openness about worries and intimate life details in some care relationships) might reflect broader differences in 'gendered' upbringing or in cultural background, but might also reflect quite small differences in individual biography, family history and mores. Deciding on the boundaries of discriminatory and non-discriminatory practices is very contentions and, once again, subject to both empirical and ideological disagreement. Our evaluation of specific social institutions will reflect our wider stances on the organisation of societies and polities as whole.

If we now turn our attention to the construction of whole health systems, or even whole health ecologies, it should be obvious *both* that the same broad issues of balancing system, group and individual interests and perspectives will inevitably arise, *and* that there can be no easy or single answer to finding such balances because systems have to address diverse purposes: they have – for example, through health promotion policies – to help to provide a collective social foundation for both individual and community development, health and well-being; and they have – for example, in clinical consultations – to be responsive to the specific agendas and preferences of diverse groups of people and individuals. But, once again, the contrasts that are being drawn here must be relative and not absolute. It is obviously not possible for health promotion or social medicine to set aside group variation and individual autonomy, nor is it possible for the clinical care of individuals to proceed effectively except in the context of a common field of action that is planned around the needs of communities and populations. I will explore these tensions and balances further by looking, in turn, at health promotion and the organisation of clinical care.

Health promotion: for populations, groups or individuals?

Perhaps the most often repeated idea that informs aspirations towards reoriented health policy is the need to focus attention beyond the one-to-one clinical encounter. Although, thankfully, doctors and other health professionals can do a great deal to treat and support people, there is a now a widespread recognition that there is lot that they cannot do, or cannot do on their own. This applies – even keeping the emphasis on the management of disease or illness – at every stage of a potential or actual illness trajectory. There are steps that might be taken to prevent illness, to improve decision making about the treatment of illness and to improve the course of living with and managing an illness that involve non-clinical actors, including not only patients and families and policy makers but many others. There are a lot of aspects of, and names for, this broader agenda but one label that is chosen by some – and that has the advantage of sounding relatively open ended – is 'health promotion'. Health promotion refers to the myriad ways in which people's physical and social environments might be made healthier, and in which opportunities can be created to help people enjoy healthier lives or contribute to the health of others. Given that more or less everything – including the economy, housing, transport, employment, education, air quality and so on – is relevant to the promotion of health, and that there are a number of competing approaches and models in health promotion, this is an immensely complex and contested field and one that it is impossible to review adequately here (Cragg et al, 2013). But it is possible, by considering an example, to indicate some of the implications, and complications, of thinking about health policy with health promotion in mind.

A policy maker or health professional interested in social action might, for example, see good grounds for seeking to reduce the levels of alcohol or sugar consumption within the communities they serve. Faced with plenty of epidemiological evidence that these things add to the total burden of disease and disability, and thereby contribute to the suffering of many of the people they seek to serve, policy makers and professionals may reasonably judge that they have a sufficient practical and moral basis to support intervention. However, any such intervention is likely to be contentious. This is not least because of the long, complex (and to some degree disputed) lines of causation that allow for multiple points of intervention with differential impacts on organisations and individuals.

How far should intervention be at a societal and structural level – such as by regulating the marketing of certain products, or perhaps reducing the availability of cheap alcohol by legislating for a minimum unit price, or introducing a 'sugar tax' as a disincentive? Or how far should interventions be aimed at specific groups or individuals, perhaps with more emphasis on 'softer' methods such as education or peer support? This question indicates the most persistent, and frequently discussed, set of dilemmas in health promotion. Where we place the emphasis is partly a pragmatic question – what are we (depending on our role) able to do, and what do we think will be effective? But it is also a question that reflects different ideological inclinations and has its own moral and political implications. Many health promoters are cautious about placing too much weight on the roles of individual actors or 'consumers'. Why locate the key responsibility with them; isn't this no more than applying a misguided 'victim blaming' attitude (Tones and Tilford, 2001)? Those who share this worry will want to investigate broader causes and more radical structural interventions. Why not, perhaps, directly intervene in the policies of those companies that make profits out of these products by, for example, restricting the production and marketing of certain products or heavily taxing company profits? Why not look more broadly at the environments and stressors that (along with marketing) encourage people to seek consolation from certain products? The focus on these consumables is – it could be asserted – already starting too far down chain of the factors that determine people's health and well-being.

It is in this context that worries and complaints about the threat of the 'nanny state' frequently arise in popular media.

Let us imagine that Leonard is one such complainer. Leonard feels very strongly that what he eats or drinks should be up to him. If he wants to buy 'unhealthy' products that is his choice. Furthermore, he can confidently assert that he is a responsible consumer who looks after himself. He eats a balanced diet, does not use very much processed food and drinks only an occasional glass of wine with his dinner and has the odd sweet for a treat. Not only does he not need to be told what to do but it is, he feels sure, completely unfair for him to be expected to pay extra through 'punitive' taxes for engaging in practices that affect no one else and that do not even impair his own health or constitute a significant risk to it. Leonard's case is indicative of the set of dilemmas referred to above. On the one hand, he seems to be advancing a reasonable argument about potential health promotion policies being insensitive to, and perhaps unfair to, him. But, on the other hand, is it reasonable for him to expect the policy climate to fully reflect his individual circumstances and preferences?

Let us imagine that living around the corner from him are Greta, a three-year old-girl, and Su, her mother. Su is supportive of some legislative intervention in this area. She is the sole carer for Greta and, naturally, worries about Greta's long-term health and well-being. She would prefer for manufacturers to be forced to put less sugar in products but, in addition or instead, she would also support a 'sugar tax'. Su knows that she and Greta eat too many sugary products and is trying to cut down, and she believes that anything that might help to rebalance the food and drink markets towards healthier products is worth trying. She worries about her own will-power to make the right choices and would value some collective intervention and message that reinforces her good intentions or some more direct local advice and support. She thinks, 'Even if it is getting a bit too late for me I would like Greta to grow up into a world that supported healthier eating choices.'

Obviously, policy makers cannot fully implement both Leonard's and Su's policy preferences. One way forward is to look for compromises that differentiate between different constituencies or sub-populations. This might include taking a much stricter line on products and marketing that seem to be directly aimed at children. This may help to protect Greta's future health while perhaps leaving Leonard relatively untroubled (of course he may still object to the 'nanny state' interfering in what he sees as purely a parental function, or he may be further annoyed if his occasional treat is a specific brand of 'children's sweets'). In addition, health promotion could be pursued as much as possible using a targeted, rather than a population, approach. This might, for example, mean offering Su, and others who are interested, various informal health-education opportunities, including invitations to a local peer-run support group or community-action initiative. The latter has some significant advantages. It is less crude than national policy measures and it may help people to address some of their concerns and habits at a deeper level, and create a genuine sense of solidarity and of being both active and supported in the process. But it may also have some disadvantages. Such grassroots provision and action can – cumulatively – be expensive, require a lot of organisation and likely end up being quite 'patchy'. And although it may provide some forms of solidarity it will not tackle Su's more general civic concerns about the bad practices of the food industry.

Ultimately, however, there is no meaningful way in which an approach oriented solely towards individuals and sub-populations – although it can make a vital contribution – can provide the whole solution either to health-promotion challenges or to public policy formulation more broadly. It simply does not make sense to imagine that the answer to the problem of finding public policy accord is for everything to be done at an individual or group level. People live within some shared framework, whether or not they wish to do so. It would be practically impossible to take Leonard's 'leave it up to individual responsibility' approach to very many things, such as air and water quality, or transport safety policies and so on. Furthermore, there is no obvious 'default' position in matters such as the regulation of the food and drinks industry. Unless anyone is allowed to produce, market and sell anything at all in any way they like – which would mean rolling back all food-safety provisions, for a start – then the central question is not whether or not to regulate for health reasons but how and where to draw the line on such regulations.

One of the differences between Leonard and Su's outlooks, as represented here, is that Leonard is stressing what he sees as his interests (and perhaps the interests of other similarly placed people) as a separate individual, whereas Su is to some extent – at least in her advocacy of structural reform of the food industry – explicitly alluding to some notion of the common good. It is important to note that there can be no presumption about which of these positions is more basic – it is simply a mistake to presume that 'individuals as separate' exist first and then social perspectives (that recognise 'individuals as inseparable') come after that. (This is the problematic presumption often labelled as 'methodological individualism'.) Rather, a central issue for social ethics is how to strike a balance between these two ways of seeing persons in the way we construct and respond to policy problems. There are certainly some health-related goods that can be approached only in collective terms. The paradigm case here is what are sometimes called 'public goods', like clean air. 'Public goods' is an expression that can be used in a restricted sense (roughly meaning goods that can be enjoyed by everyone without anyone missing out). But there are many other analogous kinds of 'common goods' or 'shared goods' relevant to public health, which are like public goods in the sense that they can effectively be planned and enacted only collectively. Su's demands for a responsible food industry and for authoritative social information, 'symbolic' messages and support for civic action directed towards healthy eating fall into this category.

In addition to arguments from the common good there are, of course, arguments for public health-oriented structural interventions that are motivated by considerations of equality. One of the clearest implications of understanding that health experiences are socially determined is the recognition that people do not have equal health opportunities – whether those be opportunities to avoid disease, to live long lives, to participate in their own healthcare or in policy formation or simply to be able to enjoy whatever health they have (Marmot, 2015; Bambra, 2016). Health promoters have long recognised that people can be in considerably stronger or weaker positions to 'look after themselves'. Forms of social disadvantage (financial, housing related, environmental, educational and so on) tend to accumulate together and reinforce one another (Wolff and De-Shalit, 2007; Graham, 2009). It follows that policies that devolve responsibility for health-related behaviour to individuals, as opposed to collectively sharing them, will have differential, and often substantially unfair, impacts. This is another crucial rationale for societal-level interventions, whether these are universal or more targeted.

There are also ethical challenges attached to the 'targeting' of interventions that have to be acknowledged. How should policy makers at national or local levels draw up inclusion and exclusion criteria? Even assuming that such health-promotion provision is successfully targeted at those who both need and value it, then how can services and professionals ensure that the selection and enactment of interventions is not discriminatory, or otherwise unfair, in the kinds of ways discussed earlier in the chapter? There are a number of substantial hazards to negotiate here. There is not only the danger of identifying certain 'at risk' groups and neglecting others, but also the danger of stigmatising the people who are targeted. If health-promotion strategies are planned without attention to the real risks of creating stigma – or anxiety, stress or social exclusion and so on – then good intentions to promote physical well-being may simply translate into the exacerbation of threats to mental well-being. If, for instance, Su were to be invited to a health-promotion programme as a local 'single parent' there is a danger that such a programme would assume and foster a deficit account of one-parent families, when there are many others (who do not fall into this category) who could be as interested in and may have as much chance of benefiting from, an intervention. In addition, there is a risk of targeting people who might benefit from certain kinds of health promotion but who have many other, including some more pressing, needs that may mean that the intended health promotion is ineffective and is experienced as marginal to people's concerns. (To put this bluntly, individuals in a similar position to Su's may well be inclined to say, 'Forget targeted support on nutrition, please just provide me with a decent minimum income and I will struggle less and be able to better contribute to my children's health and well-being in all kinds of ways.') This risk may also coincide with the risk of 'medicalising' issues that might be better dealt with as social issues (as discussed in Chapter Two), at least, that is, where narrow, biomedically defined life-style approaches dominate health-promotion practice rather than more structural or community-development approaches.

Even from this simple example it is clear that neither 'whole society' nor targeted approaches to health promotion are unproblematic. Those who argue that the individual person provides the wrong focus and places the burden of responsibility in the wrong place – expecting individual consumers to manage risks produced by big businesses and others who systematically create an environment in which healthy choices are not always easy to make – press home a vitally important point. (One that echoes the sociological critiques of choice and 'responsibilisation' set out in the last chapter.) But, as things stand, that is the environment in which Su finds herself and she would welcome some support in whatever form it comes. People sometimes want to *take* responsibility for things – including things that other people conscientiously judge that they ought not to be *held* responsible for – and that is something that surely needs to be respected and responded to constructively.

Su – along with many other people who might either seek, or potentially benefit from, targeted forms of health promotion – is in an ambivalent position. Su is effectively saying 'help me to help myself'. This suggests that it is a mistake to imagine that there is an easily identified, unified and transparent 'self' to relate to or help. People – and surely this is all of us and not some 'needy' sub-set of the population – are pulled in different directions and have conflicting desires and dispositions. This can be a messy business. It is easier to understand and analyse these situations by recognising some desires to be what have been called 'second-order desires', that is, desires about our desires (Frankfurt, 1982). We can, for example, be strongly inclined to indulge in some behaviour – such as tobacco smoking – and, at the same time, have a clear and sustained desire to resist or overcome the inclination. But, of course, it is not always that easy for us or others to confidently identify an unequivocal hierarchy between our desires and preferences. Practitioners who work with groups and individuals – whether clinicians, health promoters or peers and so on – have to manage some skilful and sensitive balancing acts. There are strong echoes here of the discussion of shared decision-making in the last chapter. Any model of shared decision-making that rests on a straightforward picture of 'preference elicitation', in which people's preferences can be extracted from them like jelly beans from a jar – separate, sharply defined and solid – is a very misleading model.

Organising clinical care

As noted in the introduction to this chapter, there are many parallels and overlaps between the social dimension of public health and the social dimension of clinical care. In both cases there are not only potential tensions between population, group and individual priorities but also tensions that arise within each level.

All clinical care is socially based. Clinical roles and relationships are not like private acts of care giving between two strangers washed up on a desert island. People who seek care from health professionals are meeting people in socially sanctioned roles who belong to professional associations and who are based in, or work for, authorised social institutions. Professionals, and the professions and institutions that legitimate them, are embedded in complex webs of accountability – to their patients or clients and local populations, to employers, to professional peers and leaders, to state agencies that recognise and monitor them and to the wider society. Given this, it is inevitable that social expectations and standards will define the field. Healthcare professionalism might even be roughly defined as about the production of, and the meeting of, expectations and standards – patients and populations need to be able to expect, and trust, that certain standards (defined in terms of both technical quality and ethics) will be met or at least striven towards (Cribb and Gewirtz, 2015).

This means that when we go to see a health professional – including on a fee-for-service model – we do not meet as abstract individuals who can simply invent our roles and working relationship, but within a socially regulated and coordinated context. Sometimes the parameters may be fairly wide, but we each have a recognised role to play and – if things are as they should be – the comparatively vulnerable patient can be reasonably confident that the person looking after them, and the treatment they are being offered, have both passed numerous tests of social acceptability. Of course, if someone is paying directly and can afford to do so, they may have chosen a particular practitioner expressly because that practitioner is somewhat idiosyncratic, or an outright maverick. But even then the same broad logic will usually apply. To be a maverick professional still implies membership of, and sufficient cohesion with, a professional community. (To choose to see someone who had been positively rejected and excluded by their professional and institutional peers would not only be rare but would take us into a completely different topic.) However, the degree of coordination and cohesion is normally quite high. Most clinical care takes place in settings that are self-consciously managed and orchestrated to achieve significant levels of consistency in provision.

As mentioned in the previous chapter, this is partly because, but not just because, the resources people spend on healthcare are often 'pooled' and this – because it is wrong to waste common resources – necessitates the productive and efficient use of resources. And efficiency suggests a certain measure of consistency; that is to say, it makes sense to offer diversity of provision only in cases where there is some significant level of relevant variation between people. Clearly, different individuals and groups will need to be treated differently, but not normally for the sake of it or on any grounds whatsoever. If the purchasing department normally buys a certain design of bed or buys a prescription medicine from a particular provider we cannot and should not expect it to alter its order just because someone has a preference for a different colour of bed or tablet that entails making an extra order or going to a new provider (Barber, 1991). In addition to 'pure' efficiency considerations there are a number of more fundamental and substantive factors that work in favour of a presumption of consistency.

Healthcare requires high levels of social coordination. Providing greater levels of variation in care than are necessary (whatever those levels are) not only demands still greater levels of organisational effort but also is an unwarranted threat to the maintenance of quality and safety regimes and habits that provide safeguards for all patients. A similar rationale applies to the provision of treatments. This is the core rationale of evidence-based healthcare. Where there is clear evidence that certain treatments work better than others, then, all else being equal, there is both a technical and an ethical imperative to provide those treatments. Obviously it is not always the case that 'all else is equal', and I will turn to some of the difficulties that this produces shortly (and again in the following chapter), but, before that, I want to underline the value of treating people consistently, where treatment is understood in its general sense.

We need to be careful not to exaggerate worries about systems and norms. As indicated earlier in the chapter, lying in the background of these worries are genuinely troubling pictures about enforced conformity and the threat of depersonalisation or dehumanisation, such as those associated with 'total institutions' or similarly totalising (or even totalitarian) discourses and practices. But, as I have been suggesting here, effective healthcare, at least outside the wholly domestic sphere, rests upon the existence of systems and some level of attention to consistency of treatment. Moreover, this is not simply a pragmatic point but is a point of principle. A concern for equality between persons must extend to a respect for the differences between people and their different identities and choices and so on. But it must also be underpinned by a commitment to ensuring that everyone has an equal chance of being acknowledged, cared for and listened to in the first place. This, very basic, sense of equality depends upon some very mundane and routine practices. Health systems and services, for example, need to keep a record of the people they are looking after and to make sure that they keep their lists, and basic data such as contact details of patients, up to date, and that they implement appointment systems and queuing systems impartially. People who are used to the health systems in the relatively affluent developed world can easily take these things for granted. Indeed it is relatively commonplace for us to complain about the associated form filling or to despair at the bureaucratic aspects of systems and institutions. But, while bureaucracy can get out of control, it should not be seen as an intrinsically bad thing. Indeed the opposite has been argued in Paul Du Gay's rightly celebrated book *In Praise of Bureaucracy* (Du Gay, 2000).

Du Gay argues that bureaucracy is not best understood as irrelevant to, or even a simple hindrance to, the ethical treatment of people as 'whole persons' but as itself embodying an ethical framework that protects and promotes the interests of persons. Those who operate within a bureaucratic ethos, and have learned to practise the corresponding dispositions, will act impartially between persons, that is, they will ensure that each person's concerns and needs have an equal chance of being taken seriously and addressed by the systems they administer. This also entails exercising their authority and judgement in a manner that is clearly independent of the various vested interests within or around systems, including the interests and preferences of politicians who are subject to pragmatic or ideological pressures that can compromise impartiality. In addition they will aspire to neutrality, or at least a studied scepticism, about the different 'visions' of the good life or good society that politicians or other would-be reformers want to apply to the system. These tendencies and aspirations will be subject to various critiques – for example, as narrowly rationalistic or as leading to a dull empiricism, or as based upon an impossible conception of neutrality and so on – but, Du Gay argues, respect for persons requires their defence. As just noted, this provides for only a very basic and 'thin' conception of ethics, equality of treatment or respect for persons. Those designing health systems need to consider other, 'thicker' or richer, accounts of what equality or respect for different persons might entail, but it would be a mistake to imagine that these thicker conceptions can replace something like this basic, bureaucratic, approach to consistency of treatment.

Indeed one of the fundamental challenges for policy makers, in balancing consistency of treatment with responsiveness to diversity, is to combine together thinner and thicker conceptions of what is required by equality and respect for persons. This is addressed to some extent by a division of labour between, on the one hand, the administrators charged with organising systems and institutions, who for the most part can deal with only abstractly defined and categorised groups and individuals and, on the other hand, front-line professionals who meet with people in all of their complexity and who are called upon to, and have the relevant expertise to, make and defend subtle discriminations between their needs. But there is certainly no sharp division of labour here: the databases of administrators may also be designed to facilitate defensible variations in treatments; and professionals, who are increasingly actively involved in or implicated in institutional management, are mindful of the need for system-level consistency. (I will be exploring this in more depth in the next section of this chapter.) These kinds of divisions of labour can help with the practical management of, but certainly do not eliminate, the tensions between the different senses of, and 'layers' of, equal respect for persons in both their commonalities and differences. The case for basic consistency of treatment needs to be continuously balanced against the importance of justified differentiation.

Healthcare is just as subject to the risks of institutional discrimination (as well as direct discrimination) as the other social institutions – the army or the university – discussed near the start of the chapter. Obviously, in a health system where the chance of being treated or the range and quality of care options available to patients is partly a function of their spending resources or their levels of insurance coverage there is every chance that health services will serve only to manifest or exacerbate wider social inequalities. This is, for example, what has put the fairness of the US system, where millions of people have historically been without adequate insurance cover, under the spotlight. But there are equally risks of significant levels of institutional discrimination in systems where there are conscientious attempts to base provision purely on people's needs or ability to benefit from treatment – such as is the official aspiration of the UK NHS.

Designing and providing an equitable healthcare system that is sensitive to individual and social difference is fraught with challenges. For example, a minority ethnic group may be systematically disadvantaged in a range of ways: they may experience different patterns of illness to a majority ethnic group (and thus sometimes have services skewed against their needs); they may face language or other communication barriers in institutions that reflect majority cultures. These factors can produce unequal risks of over-diagnosis or under-diagnosis; prevention or health-education messages, and the assumptions underlying them, may be insensitive to different cultural norms or social circumstances; research about 'what works' that underlies many of these things can be insufficiently sensitive to these variations, and so forth. Analogous issues can arise on the basis of gender, class or other axes of social difference. All of this means that arguments about impartiality and about the merits of a basic consistency of treatment, while important, do not take us very far. Once we move beyond the abstract call for equality and get into the practice of implementation, then policy makers, service planners, managers and professionals will, in reality, be constantly navigating between competing considerations, or 'squaring circles', that is, steering narrow, and sometimes impossibly difficult, paths between different kinds of potentially justified and unjustified forms of discrimination.

The costs of efficiency

I have been arguing that there is no simple or neat contradiction between looking at things from a systems perspective and the valuing of individuals. Indeed, as we have seen, effective systems planned around the needs of populations are necessary to the delivery of equal treatment of persons. But, at the same time, there are also ongoing tensions between population perspectives and the potentially different needs and interests of sub-populations and individuals. In this final section I want to return to the idea that systems thinking will inevitably 'fall short' when it comes to the needs of individuals. This is the worry, rehearsed at the start of the chapter, about systems and institutions having a tendency to be depersonalising. In a nutshell, this worry arises because systems work on *quantitative and instrumental* logics but personal well-being also depends upon *qualitative and relational* logics (this way of putting it arises from Habermas' account of systems, which we will turn to shortly).

This book began with the observation that health systems have to provide both 'health' and 'care' and I was using the idea of 'care' there as a very rough marker not only for compassion but for the other non-instrumental dimensions of respect including recognition and inclusion. As noted before, being 'attended to' and not neglected is a fundamental good in this regard. This kind of good, by its very nature, needs to be enacted by persons and through personal relationships. A fair system will give every individual an equal chance of receiving this basic kind of recognition, and failures here can amount to important forms of inequality. This is because – as elucidated by Fraser's (1996) account, cited above – while inequalities can take the form of differences in opportunities for, or in the achievement of, health outcomes, they can also simply take the form of different experiences of being cared for, noticed or recognised, or of inclusion in meaningful dialogue and forms of participation. The latter are, of course, important supports to mental well-being but they are also of intrinsic ethical importance.

One very widespread driver behind threats to the recognition of, and care for, persons within healthcare institutions is the pressure towards system and institutional efficiency understood in instrumental terms. These threats can be understood in common-sense terms, and they can be explored in more depth by reference to the widespread critiques of both 'marketisation' and 'managerialism' in healthcare. They can also be illuminated and understood, at an even more general and theoretical level, by drawing upon Habermas' analysis of the rationalising effects of systems (Habermas, 1987). I will say something more about each of these in turn.

Everyone recognises that health services, especially in settings where there are – for whatever reasons – sustained pressures towards cost containment, can produce environments in which staff are under considerable stress because of intensification of demands and activity. And, given that healthcare often involves important 'tasks' that require effort and attention – including cognitive tasks like diagnosis, or specialised or basic practical tasks – then there is obviously a risk that the less instrumental and well-defined, and more diffuse, issue of 'relating to people' can be relatively eclipsed. This worry arises in a variety of forms, and especially within economically stretched systems or institutions. For example, it is sometimes said that staff are simply 'too busy' to pause and talk; or that space and time constraints make anything more than perfunctory exchanges impossible; or that staff are worn down or even 'burned out', and perhaps lacking the moral and emotional support that they themselves need in order to have the resources and resilience required to reach out to other people. Of course these concerns are not universal and people will equally well report experiences of having good and highly valued relationships with health professionals even in pressured environments. Nor is there, in principle, any reason why the systematisation of healthcare should marginalise caring in its various aspects – a counselling service renowned for its successful relationship-building work could well be, and is likely to be, organised very systematically.

But, although systems highly geared towards overall efficiency can support care, there are arguments worth considering that suggest that broad social changes make this, as a matter of fact, less likely. These arguments arise from critiques of both 'marketisation' and 'managerialism'. I am using these terms here as rough analogues of 'medicalisation'. In other words, I am not questioning the potential contribution of some forms of market provision or bureaucratic management to health-related goods and services (indeed I have explicitly asserted the opposite in earlier comments) but am just reflecting concerns that it is possible for either of these things to get 'out of hand' by being applied in ways, or in areas, where they do harm rather than good. (Of course people will passionately disagree about where these boundaries are, but almost everyone will agree that there are limits to be drawn in this regard.) The basic argument can be crudely summed up by saying that socioeconomic and public policy changes have systematically and increasingly blurred the division of labour between those whose role it is to ensure that institutions work efficiently and those whose role it is to be responsive to the needs of persons and, in particular, that the latter are increasingly being required to adopt the mindset of the former. More and more practitioners are being required to think of their work in terms of budget management, productivity, performance measures or similar. This phenomenon can be seen, and critiqued, as a product of an ever-growing bureaucracy with professionals subject to more and more rationalisation, including ever more finely grained 'hoops' to jump through (Germov, 2005). Or it can sometimes be presented as an unwelcome side-effect of certain kinds of market practices in which healthcare is turned into a product where every element is institutionally defined, packaged, costed and seen through the lens of the difference it makes to 'the bottom line' (McKee and Stuckler, 2012).

In many respects it makes little difference whether it is managerialism or marketisation (or some combination) that is 'blamed' for the risks to the practices, cultures and professional subjectivities of healthcare. The underlying process is one in which institutional agendas, which involve the quantification and monitoring of healthcare practices (to ensure institutional effectiveness and efficiency), become culturally dominant. This can happen, for example, when this institutional quantification helps to frame, or becomes a major feature in, the mental landscape of healthcare professionals. There are myriad ways in which this happens – through audits, clinical governance, devolved budgets, performance management and so forth. There is also a clear explanation, and an understandable and plausible rationale, for these processes. These institutions operate in environments where competition or institutional comparison exert considerable pressure, and it therefore makes sense to harness the loyalty and professional commitment of staff to ensuring that their institutions survive, or ideally thrive, despite these pressures. Thus, to repeat, this process of increasing the alignment between institutional goals and professional practices makes sense up to a point, but there is also much lively concern and criticism from those who think that it may, too often, move beyond that point. These critiques (as with the critiques of medicalisation) have been produced from different vantage points and in different genres. For example, as well as critiques of the commodification of healthcare and the oft-discussed peril of focusing too much on the measurable rather than the intangible aspects of provision, there has been extensive discussion of whether or not the 'special' nature of the professional–patient relationship can be preserved when professionals are overly subject to institutional regimes (Gilbert, 2005). The latter concern can be expressed simply – will patients cease to trust that the professional they see is interested in doing the best for them rather than in doing whatever is best for institutional or system drivers? But it cannot be so simply resolved, because there are, as we have seen in this chapter, clearly relevant considerations that support either side of this crude dichotomy.

The fundamental worry is that broader sets of social processes are somehow undermining, or positively corroding, some of the core elements of healthcare. If we take this analysis seriously it suggests that well-known examples of bad practice, including scandals about very poor care, should not automatically be treated as exceptional, but that we should be mindful that they may be symptoms of a much wider but more subtle malaise. This kind of debate surfaced to a significant extent within the UK NHS in the light of the Francis Inquiry Report into the very poor care experienced by groups of patients at Mid Staffordshire NHS Foundation Trust (HMSO, 2013). The Francis Inquiry Report did not direct the responsibility or blame solely towards the immediate health professionals or managers in the institution delivering the poor care. Rather, it very much presented it as a product of system-level cultures and practices, in particular those that sought to drive through institutional 'targets' with insufficient thought about broader consequences. This analysis informed a welcome – albeit a bleak and soul-searching – reappraisal of the emphasis that UK health policy had attached to institutional targets. In that context Mid Staffordshire and a number of other sites of analogous concern were, rightly, treated as 'outliers' but not as wholly exceptional – rather, they could be seen as indicative of a more pervasive risk to the general quality of provision across the system. The possibility I am considering here is that the issues the Francis Inquiry Report responds to and tackles might themselves be seen as no more than one example of much broader and deeper currents that transcend the specifics of the UK NHS or any one particular policy regime or approach to the running of institutions.

These deep and broad currents are characterised by Habermas (1987) as the 'colonisation' of the 'life-world' by 'systems'. Here he is obviously using language in an academic and theoretically loaded way but, I would argue, he is also illuminating and explaining contemporary social change in ways that have broad practical relevance and that reflect and amplify much in the critiques of healthcare managerialism and marketisation. Habermas is one of many social theorists who have sought to analyse and open up the complexity of the social world, and in particular how the social world both shapes and is shaped by the frameworks through which we think and act. He draws upon contrasting traditions in social thought that focus on different aspects of the social world – for example, on the one hand, large-scale, impersonal social systems – such as economic and political systems – that seek to organise and allocate goods and social positions; and on the other hand, what might be called the 'frameworks of meaning' through which we live, including cultural and personal values and identifications, that reflect and express the full range of what matters to people. Habermas' concern in talking about 'the colonisation of the life-world' is that our social life is becoming overly framed by systems – with the quantitative and instrumental logic of systems increasingly intruding into and displacing the qualitative and relational logic of people's 'life-worlds'.

Functioning societies, for Habermas, depend not only upon 'instrumental' forms of action and rationality but also on what he calls 'communicative' forms – without the latter, vital processes that underpin both mutual understanding and social legitimacy will be missing. As individuals we need to be able to get things done, but we also need to be able to relate to one another – to be able to understand, explore and negotiate things with one another. (This is broadly analogous to the insights that we have encountered before in relation to the importance of people being 'attended to' and not neglected and in relation to the importance of 'recognition' as a core dimension of equal treatment.) Yes, as a society we need social, political and economic institutions that 'work', that deliver 'outcomes', but these, if they are to be sustained and to have legitimacy, need to support communicative action and rationality. That is, they need to leave room for, and to be subject to, the perspectives and values of, and civic influence of, the people that make them work and that they are meant to serve. The fundamental problem is that the logic of systems, in Habermas' sense, is blind and unresponsive to key aspects of communicative rationality. Economic and political systems can function in many ways without the need to take mutual dialogue or deliberation seriously – there can, for example, be winners and losers, or relative success and failure, based on the counting of money or votes (or on some other quantitative indicator of economic or political power). But, as Habermas argues, if we side-line mutual understanding for the sake of system efficiency both the ultimate point of systems and the possibilities for rethinking social life are eroded.

For current purposes it is not important to defend or further elucidate Habermas' broader intellectual projects. Other commentators make closely analogous points to Habermas' from different intellectual traditions and using different vocabularies. For example, Alasdair MacIntyre makes a useful distinction between what he calls 'external goods' and 'internal goods' (MacIntyre, 2007) – the former being goods that can to a large extent be pursued instrumentally and detached from the contexts in which they arise and the latter being goods that are intrinsic or internal to the practices and contexts in which they arise. I can earn money and achieve social status including 'celebrity', for example, in a variety of different ways. These are 'external goods' because they can each to a large extent be treated as the same 'commodity' – money, status or fame – that I could attain in very different ways. But I cannot be a good chess player, a good cook or a good teacher (and so on) without entering into a specific range of practices, each with their own internal goods. If I were to attain external goods through these activities these would, crucially, not coincide with the internal goods that attach to these practices. If someone were to conflate the external and internal goods attached to an area – especially an area like teaching or caring, where the internal goods are at least partly about relationships – we could say that they simply fail to understand the nature of the area and the related practices. (We would likely feel sorry for them, and for a very good reason.) Systems can allocate external goods, but internal goods can be achieved only by people immersing themselves in activities that they, and others, experience as worthwhile (these often being demanding activities).

Health systems deal with goods that can be treated as external or internal. A number of writers have, for example, chosen to describe the forms of worthwhile activity and fulfilment that attach to the role and practices of medicine and nursing as involving internal goods (Sellman, 2011; Toon, 2014), and similar points could also be made about the practices of families, friends and patients who subject themselves to the disciplines of 'caring' or 'self-management'. But the goods of healthcare can also be treated as 'external' ones and this happens to the extent that our thinking is dominated by such ideas as 'outputs' or 'productivity'. 'Outputs' are obviously very important. But if health policy is looked at only through this lens, something seriously harmful happens to healthcare.

Conclusion

This chapter started from the presumption that anti-reductionist or holistic currents in health policy are to be welcomed. Nothing I have said is meant to argue against that. What I have been concerned to do is to underline the level of complexity and contestability that is generated by the various possible interpretations of 'holism'. As with the previous chapter, the point is that this level of contestability is not, in essence, a product of a shortage of empirical knowledge or technical know-how. Of course more and better research and logistical capacity could, as ever, make an important contribution to tackling the related difficulties. But, ultimately, disagreements about combating or counter-balancing reductionism are philosophical disputes about the nature of healthcare and the shape of the good society. I began by highlighting one possible set of contests – the tensions between individuals and social systems or institutions. Signalling the dilemmas this gives rise to, and especially the difficult question of what a concern for (the various dimensions of) equality would entail in this context, has, hopefully, served to indicate some of the challenges faced by reforming health policies. But the fact that it is complex does not mean that it is impossible to come to any tentative conclusions about what matters. For example, it seems that it would be difficult to insist on an (unrefined) 'individuals come first' position, not least because, as I have argued, both equality and 'individual respect' depend upon a high degree of social organisation. More generally, personal health and well-being depend upon common goods, including public goods.

Nonetheless, there does seem to be an important residual worry – a worry with which I opened and closed the chapter – about certain versions of 'systems thinking' leading to a serious risk to persons;

specifically, the risk of depersonalisation or dehumanisation My argument here – which came to the fore in the closing section – is that this risk does not arise directly from the relationships between individuals and groups (or populations) but, rather – following Habermas – from two different ways of conceiving of that relationship. The individual–group relationship can be constructed both as a causal/instrumental one and as a communicative/co-constitutive one. On this account the risk of depersonalisation stems from the latter being marginalised by the former. In other words, and to echo the earlier discussion about choice, persons need to be conceived of relationally – they can be treated as 'separable' entities for some purposes, but it is a mistake to see this as reflecting their fundamental nature. I should stress that the concern about this form of depersonalisation is not just a theoretical one. It is a very real risk as policy actors (nationally, locally and institutionally) press for constant 'efficiency gains'. On the face of it, the parallel ascendancy of policy discourses about 'personalisation' might provide some protection from these risks. That is the subject of the next chapter.

FIVE

Especially for you

One of the most important ideas shaping health-policy reform and debate is 'personalisation'. (Albeit, as we will see in this chapter, it is probably more accurate not to think of personalisation as one idea but as a collection of overlapping ideas and discourses.) In many ways personalisation is emblematic of the issues discussed across the book as a whole. In contemporary social life there is an expectation that people will not only want to shape and create their own lives and identities but that they will want to do so in ways that reflect, and contribute to, their individuality. This has become an intensely powerful, albeit often unexamined, norm associated, for example, both with consumer values and identity politics. Indeed some might quickly dismiss its pervasiveness as an expression of a mindless consumerism or as an absurd preoccupation with identity. But – although, as discussed in Chapter Two, we should be ready to be sceptical about currents of individualised 'self-making' – we cannot afford to be completely dismissive of this norm because it can also be seen, at least on some credible interpretations, as having an important ethical dimension. Taylor (1992) has captured this in his analysis of the ethics of authenticity: in summary, if our actions and commitments, including the choices we make, are to be serious, and to be worth taking seriously by others, it makes sense that they are genuine expressions of who we each are and where we each stand.

In a consumerist context the language of personalisation gets used in connection with almost every kind of commodity or service. A quick Google search uncovers a vast number of personalised products – T-shirts, number plates, mugs, phone cases and chocolates. It also quickly becomes evident that the same term is applied to a range of less tangible goods such as interior design or funerals. The idea of personalisation is clearly a powerful resource for marketing or branding purposes, or more generally for promoting or legitimating activities. In every case something deemed valuable is being sold or otherwise signalled through the use of the term.

It seems that the key idea and value here – and the one I will concentrate on in this chapter – is that the good in question is 'tailored to' or 'fitted to' the person in question. This, in itself, would be a sufficient reason for claiming some 'added value' over a 'common or garden' good. But there are other, looser associations of the broad idea that a good is being 'made personal' that can reinforce the positive connotations of the term. These are worth acknowledging briefly here, not just because they contribute in some vague way to the positive charge of the language of personalisation, but also because there are occasions where they have direct relevance to the appraisal of personalisation policies. 'Personal' connects to the idea of uniqueness or specific individuality – and hence to what I am treating as the core sense of personalisation as 'tailoring' – but it can also connect to other fundamentally important ideas such as intimacy or privacy. If a service is to be personal to me then I might expect that it deals with me not just confidentially but with sensitivity and delicacy – perhaps in the way I might only normally be treated by a friend. In addition I might expect to be treated as a private and separate individual, that is, not through a service that everyone and anyone knows about and uses, or is able to gain benefit from. In both these cases personalisation can have connotations of 'specialness' or exclusivity – here we might think about the contrast between a personal letter and a circular letter, or between a personal or private car, jet or boat and public forms of transport. These broader connotations also resonate with the central idea of 'individual tailoring' – if something is carefully designed to suit me, that will necessitate an element of 'intimate attention' or invasiveness in order to elicit the relevant personal data to inform its design, and if it is meant specifically for me it is not, by definition, meant for anyone else.

This chapter will, in its general storyline, echo those of the previous two chapters. Whilst acknowledging the value of personalisation as a dimension of a more person-centred healthcare I will, at the same time, seek to underline the complications and challenges that discourses of personalisation generate. Once again, that is, I want to argue that an idea that is sometimes simply presented as part of the solution might be better seen as a useful way of opening up new puzzles – in particular puzzles about competing visions of healthcare provision. As with 'choice' and 'holism' – the foci of the two previous chapters – personalisation is a concept that can gain widespread assent. It points in the general direction of something valuable, but it also accommodates a significant degree of open-endedness; that is, personalisation can encompass a very broad range of ideas, practices and values. For that reason it provides a useful banner under which to build the kinds of consensus needed to give policy making relevance and appeal. But this same conceptual, practical and ideological elasticity can serve to disguise significant divergences in the way the idea of personalisation is interpreted or applied (Cribb and Owens, 2010). In the following section I will present an introductory overview of these divergences and in the remainder of the chapter I will follow up a few of these in greater depth.

All things to all people

Depending upon how it is interpreted, personalisation can be presented as contributing to both medicalising and de-medicalising currents of healthcare change. It can be used to refer to closer attention and responsiveness to individual biology – an advancement or extension of the biomedical model. And it can be used to refer to closer attention and responsiveness to individual biography – something complementary to, or sometimes disruptive of, the biomedical model. I will rely on a very rough distinction between 'personalised medicine' and 'personalised care' to indicate this difference of emphasis.

Of course it should be said that there is nothing new about individualising or tailoring healthcare. It would no doubt be rare to find either a contemporary or a historical practitioner who would not claim to be doing this in some sense. Unless you are literally a subscriber to the notion that you can offer a panacea – a universal remedy – then you will be offering people the treatments that 'match' their conditions and needs. Clinical healthcare, unlike some aspects of population or public health, is always already 'targeted' healthcare. But both technological and cultural changes mean that possibilities and expectations of the degree of 'tailoring' – to people's bodies, on the one hand, or to people's values and/or life circumstances, on the other – have substantially expanded and intensified. (Here I am deliberately signalling a further degree of open-endedness *within* the notion of personalised care – the tension between interpreting 'biography' to stress the 'internal world' of individuals (values and preferences and so on) or the 'external world' (social circumstances), noting that these two are not discrete in any tidy sense.)

I will come back to the possible tensions between what I am calling personalised medicine and personalised care throughout the chapter, but before that I will continue to review some other dimensions of variation between versions of personalisation. Even from the very short discussion thus far some of the variations are clear. On the one hand, we can emphasise the very specific combinations of characteristics that apply to a unique individual. On the other hand, personalisation can be a matter of degree. More or less broad-brush or fine-grained differentiations between people can be made because individuals share the characteristics of broader or narrower groups. This applies whether we are thinking in terms of biological (for example, genetic) categories or more psychosocial or social categories (for example, being relatively risk averse or belonging to a particular religious community). Again, this spectrum is familiar from the retail market – there has been a huge proliferation of product variation, and clothes, for example, can be wholly bespoke or they can come in a few standard sizes or with very many permutations (not just size, but fabric, patterns and features) which give people a sense of product personalisation.

There are also variations in relation to the matter of who 'does' the personalising. Is it done by someone else – the 'expert fitter' – or is it done by the person themselves exercising their own agency, or perhaps by parties in combination? This issue does not coincide neatly with the distinction between personalised medicine and personalised care. A professional can aim for personalised care either by making their own judgements, based on relevant data, about what 'fits with' the life circumstances and life projects of a patient and/or by asking the patient to articulate or explore options and make choices.

Part of the power of the language of personalisation is that it has strong resonances with a range of ethical and political values. It is, not least, compatible with ideologies broadly of the left and the right. For those within social movements that question professional authority and orthodoxies, personalisation can represent both greater equality and 'empowerment' from paternalism or exclusionary practices. For example, those within the disability movement have sometimes embraced the idea of personalisation – as manifest in strategies like devolved personal budgets to enable people to purchase personal assistance (among other things) – as a chance to organise their health and social care in ways that are more sensitive to their own lives, circumstances, values and priorities and better insulated from medical or state paternalism or oppression. Yet these very same practices – of getting a budget to purchase what one thinks best from the marketplace, including becoming an employer of an assistant – can also be read as the marketisation of care and an extension of neoliberal logic (Mladenov et al, 2015).

This example also indicates the variety of kinds of practices that might be described as 'personalising' – these do not just include 'high tech' tailoring of diagnostic techniques or treatments, but can include very different things such as individual care planning or personal budgets. This follows from the generality and elasticity of the idea and the fact that different agents might take a lead, or participate, in the process, with the result that there are many possible axes and aspects

– for example, genetic, biochemical, genetic, emotional, social and financial – of personalisation. One very broad distinction between axes of personalisation that I will just mention here, but which I will come back to in a later section, is the one between what might be labelled causal and communicative approaches to personalisation. This overlaps with the distinction between personalised medicine and personalised care, in that the former stresses the possible variations in the causal pathways that determine biological, including disease processes, whereas the latter can stress the variations in the life-worlds, cultures, character dispositions and priorities of people, who may therefore need 'relating to' in different ways. (The overlap is not complete both because I want to use the idea of personalised care to contain the possibility of (causally) intervening in social circumstances, and because it is possible to take a causal approach to communication.) What I particularly wish to note here – and will return to at the end of the chapter – is the potential for personalisation to be linked to non-instrumental communication. In other words, I want to flag up the possibility of thinking of personalisation as occurring when individual voices and narratives are heard and acknowledged, whether or not this results in further 'outputs' for the system or for the person concerned.

To sum up, personalisation can apply to processes either side of conventional dichotomies, such as the 'objective' body and the 'subjective' life project, or 'off the peg' or bespoke consumption, or care for individuals versus choice by individuals. But it is also bound up with social and technological changes that cross and blur these dichotomies. These days, bodies can be life projects, the distinction between off the peg and bespoke is less clear cut, and the rise and advocacy of co-production is about building bridges between care and choice.

This brief overview, considered alongside the ground covered in the last two chapters, indicates some of the key dilemmas that arise in interpreting and applying aspirations for personalisation. Most obviously there is the question of how to decide when a demand for personalisation stops being a reasonable request to have one's distinctive needs met and starts to become an unreasonable expectation of 'special treatment', where this implies wastefulness or direct unfairness. More broadly, there is the question of whether, and how far, personalisation practices might be used to combat inequalities (by, for example, strengthening the position of otherwise disadvantaged people) or whether and when the underlying logic of personalisation – at least in its consumerist manifestations – simply reinforces competitive individualism and market inequalities. In short, there are big questions about the relationship between the influence of discourses of personalisation and health equity. I will touch on these from time to time in this chapter, however, for the most part I will be focusing on the question about the nature of personalisation already introduced, namely, what aspect of 'persons' can and should personalisation reflect? As I have stressed already, this is a far too wide-ranging agenda to review fully here and I will simply offer short accounts of three indicative and contrasting faces of personalisation: the arrival of personalised medicine, personalisation as enabled by devolved personal budgets and personalised care planning and attention.

Personalised medicine: new frontiers and new challenges

The arrival of personalised medicine is often described in dramatic terms. Commentators sometimes talk about a 'new era' or 'new paradigm' of healthcare or use a similar 'transformational' language. This dramatic, and sometimes sensationalist, tone is a common feature of all scientific and technological advances that carry hopes and fears with them. It is all too easy either to be carried along by promising expectations or to dismiss them as hype. However, it is clear already that personalised medicine represents something more than a simple – minor or major – technological advance. It connects to a general reorientation of biomedical thinking and practice based upon a substantial growth in knowledge of the constitution of people's bodies. Specifically, as it has become increasingly possible to 'zoom in' on the detailed constitution of individual people's biology, then the understanding of the possibilities of tailoring care to individuals has grown, as has insight into its potential benefits.

Originally the language of personalised medicine was mainly used in connection with the genetic variations between people. The fact that each person has a unique genetic make-up, combined with the ability to sequence an individual's full set of genes or genome, has led to the capacity to design and apply treatments or diagnostic tests more sensitively. For example, genetic testing can help to increase the chance that some HIV+ patients will respond well to certain treatments and help to steer prescribers towards some drugs rather than others. The recognition that people's genetic constitution can influence their level of susceptibility to certain diseases or the way they respond to interventions produces the potential for an indefinitely large number of new medical interventions. Although most of these hypothetical interventions still exist at an 'in principle' rather than 'in practice' level there are some examples that have become well established and known, such as the potential to apply genetic testing for an increased risk of breast cancer, which then creates opportunities for women with positive tests to, for example, get earlier or more regular breast screening (NIH National Cancer Institute, 2016).

More recently the term 'personalised medicine' has come to be applied more broadly than to genetic medicine. The same major technological developments that have led to progress in genetics – the abilities to work at a cellular and molecular level and to quickly compute enormous quantities of data – have led to the capacity to identify and make use of a broad range of biological markers or 'biomarkers' – not just genes but, for example, the presence of specific biochemical entities, molecules or biological processes – to assess the risks, presence or trajectory of a disease, or the effects or possible impacts of treatment options in diverse individuals. This makes it possible to target disease processes more precisely – for example, by differentiating between tumour types or distinct underlying biochemical pathways – and hence this movement is sometimes referred to as 'precision medicine'. (Increasingly the terms 'personalised' or 'precision medicine' are being deployed to refer to the use of the vast range of computable data about individuals – including biological and non-biological data, such as life-style-related data –to inform medicine.)

These technological developments are subject to various controversies, some of which I will simply note here because, even though they are both important and interesting, they are not my primary focus. Noting these controversies is not intended to sound dismissive of the promise of personalised medicine. They do no more than indicate what might be expected – that significant promises are accompanied by significant threats. A major area of concern is evident in the example of genetic testing for breast screening just mentioned. The way in which personalised medicine might shed light on people's susceptibility to future disease means that advocates will often highlight its potential contribution to shifting the balance of healthcare from treatment to prevention. But, even assuming that this potential could be systematically realised in reliable ways, this obviously produces new sets of social and ethical challenges. When, and how far, is it really helpful for people to be able to 'see into the future' by being given an account of their risk profile or their chances of responding to treatment? Given that the data used is digitised and instantly transmitted via the internet or stored in the cloud for long periods of time, is it practically possible to protect the resulting data sets and analyses so as to ensure privacy? How might the fact that this kind of information exists affect people's access to insurance? These kinds of questions, and the concerns lying behind them, are sufficient to illustrate that the benefits offered by personalised medicine are not cost or risk free and require public scrutiny (Nuffield Council on Bioethics, 2010).

More fundamentally, it is possible to view personalised medicine as representing an extension and intensification of medicalisation; in other words, to see the movement as exacerbating the worries discussed in Chapter Two – for example, the dangers of interpreting people's lives and life fortunes too heavily in biomedical categories, including conceiving of health and well-being largely through reductionist lenses, or over-reliance on scientific and technical 'fixes'. In particular, the intensification of the focus that is inherent in personalised medicine makes substantial demands on people – it is potentially highly intrusive or invasive, requiring new levels of surveillance and access to data, and resource intensive, in so far as interventions will sometimes require 'bespoke' research or production of interventions. In addition, the possibility of identifying an ever-multiplying number of 'risk factors' not only greatly increases the chances of over-diagnosis and over-treatment but creates many new kinds of potential 'sickness identities' – more or less substantial – for people to assume and worry about. There is also, of course, the potential to reinforce or significantly increase health inequalities, at least inequalities of access to this form of high-tech medicine.

On the other hand, it is quite possible to present personalised medicine as creating many more opportunities for people – and not just for doctors, researchers and public and private organisations but for citizens, in collectives or as individuals, who can be put in a position of having greater access to data and technology to research, self-monitor and participate in their own healthcare. Specifically, personalised medicine policies should not be seen as something wholly 'done by' some and 'done to' others. (This is further considered in Chapter Seven.) All of the discussions in earlier chapters – and more generally embedded in health-policy discourses – about the need for partnership and for operating with a broad conception of 'health actors' have relevance here. There is a need for community and civic engagement with debates about personalised medicine and there is, as ever, an imperative for patients and families who are, or may be, implicated in specific developments to be able to exercise their agency in concert with one another and to be able to help determine what happens to them by embracing some opportunities and resisting others. In this connection some policy analysts prefer to use an idea like 'policy enactment' rather than 'policy implementation' to stress that policies are not necessarily 'made' in one place (in authoritative bodies) and 'delivered' in others (on the ground). Policy enactment theory highlights the multi-directional nature of policy action. It rejects the assumption that policy is one directional – operating from centres of power outwards, and created by some and 'implemented' by others; and analyses policy as something constantly being made and remade, inflected, contested and disrupted at every stage, level and context by indefinitely large numbers of people (Ball et al, 2011). Not everyone is equally well placed to shape what happens but the mix of influence is not an 'all or nothing' dichotomy, and is itself something that can be attended to and shaped. However, there are reasons to be concerned – on current trajectories – about the balance between the level of patient and public 'contribution' to personalised data sets and the level of 'control' that patients and publics have over the use of such data sets or, more generally, over the policy direction and practices of personalised medicine (Prainsack, 2017).

This discussion of dispersed agency brings to a head some of the ambiguity in the notion of personalisation. The typical meaning of 'personalised' contained within the term 'personalised medicine' is responsiveness to an individual's biology. Whereas within broader discourses of person–centred care personalisation might typically be taken to refer to responsiveness to an individual's life circumstances and/ or their wishes or choices. At a prosaic everyday level this ambiguity might entail, for example, that clinicians and their patients sometimes have different things in mind when they hear about or talk about treatment being personalised. This possibility is significant in its own right and I will turn to it in a moment. But obviously, lying behind this, there are deeper questions – not least about the business of holding divergent senses of personalisation together – that constitute the main concern of this chapter.

Sarah Denford and colleagues have investigated the different interpretations that can be given to the personalisation or 'individualisation' of drug treatment by doctors and patients, and within the literature (2013, 2014). Their work is based on literature review and relatively small-scale qualitative interviewing and does not claim to represent populations but, rather, to illuminate different possible interpretations of concepts. It is also not focused on personalised medicine per se, in the specific sense used in this section, but it is set in the context of personalised medicine. It is thus helpful in illuminating the 'baseline' conceptions of personalisation on the ground. In the case of the people they spoke to there was a range of emphases from doctors – with some primarily stressing doctor-led and evidence-based personalisation and others giving some weight to responsiveness to patients' priorities. In their interviews with doctors comparatively few of them referred to the scope to support patients to personalise treatments after the consultation. By contrast, in their discussions with patients who were active in a 'patient and public involvement' (PPI) group emphasis was given to the capacity for patients to help tailor their own treatments through 'trial and error', albeit within parameters of safety set by, and drawing upon advice and information from, their doctors.

Denford et al conclude that terms such as personalisation and individualisation are used – within the literature they reviewed and the people they spoke to – in very inconsistent and sometimes contradictory ways. In some instances, for example, patient involvement was highlighted yet, at the same time, 'the "patient's perspective" was completely absent from much of the literature purporting to be about individualisation (e.g. pharmacogenetics)' (Denford et al, 2014). Denford et al argue for the potential of what they label MAT or 'mutually agreed tailoring'. This is a version of the forms of partnership working discussed in Chapter Three (roughly a combination of shared decision-making and support for self-management). But the difficulties of this kind of working are also recognised, including by the members of the PPI group:

> The group recognised limitations to this description of individualisation. It was noted that not all patients want their treatments to be individualised in this way. Second, patients described the considerable level of involvement required of the patient. It was acknowledged that not all patients will be motivated to make such an effort. Third, with this approach comes the potential for patients to be left feeling unsupported. Finally, the group recognised that individualisation of treatment is challenging (if not impossible) without continuity of care. (Denford et al, 2013, Introduction)

These reflections from patients reinforce the concerns rehearsed earlier about shared decision-making, especially where this is interpreted as 'transferring responsibility' to patients. Responsibility, especially without corresponding support, is a burden that not all patients are equally well placed to take or interested in assuming.

In summary, personalised medicine – where this is understood largely in terms of responsiveness to individual biology – creates many opportunities to make biomedicine more responsive to human variation, including individual variation, and thereby to make interventions more effective. It also presents a range of challenges for person-centred care understood more broadly. It might be even be viewed as an additional threat to the anti-reductionist or 'whole person' dimension of person-centredness. It gives rise to related ambiguities about the role of patient agency or patient preferences in personalisation, and how these might be integrated with biological responsiveness, while at the same time it potentially makes very significant demands on people to participate (directly or indirectly) in data-generating and analysing activities. And it can also be seen as creating new risks of, and new forms of, health inequality, either because people will have different levels of motivation or capacity to engage with personalisation processes or because their life circumstances will produce very different levels of access to relevant resources and opportunities.

Personalisation as consumption: using one's own budget

Personalised medicine creates new opportunities for the consumption of healthcare goods and services. It is now possible, for example, for individuals to buy genetic-profiling services and advice from private sector providers. But, of course, the link between the idea of 'personalisation' and individual consumption is quite independent from, and predates the language of, personalised medicine. As highlighted in previous chapters, the culture of consumerism now shapes all aspects of social life, including healthcare. And, as noted at the start of this chapter, personalisation has itself become a key trend and value in contemporary consumption.

In all health economies a substantial part of explicitly health-related expenditure flows from the private decisions of individuals. This includes such things as the 'fitness' sector (for example, fitness equipment, gym membership and personal trainers), vitamins and food supplements, and over-the-counter remedies and medicines. There is also a large 'fee for service' or 'private medicine' sector, even in systems where healthcare resources are typically pooled, so that people can, for instance, obtain access to quicker consultations or treatments or can obtain interventions that are not covered by insurance schemes or single-payer systems.

People in relatively wealthy economies take it for granted that they can use whatever spending power they have to obtain goods and services that suit them. In short, much personalisation is achieved through individual consumption patterns. Even though there is a lot of political contestation about the best way to draw and regulate the boundaries between private and collective forms of healthcare provision, most people do not question the importance of allowing some measure of individual freedom in this area. There are in any case fuzzy lines between what might count as 'healthcare' and what might be better described as 'life-style', 'leisure' or 'aesthetic' considerations. This means that even those of a strongly collectivist mind-set (such as advocates of the UK NHS) would typically be quite reluctant to rule out a place for private consumption in the health sector. In a climate where I am happy to accept that people will spend money on cosmetics, on what basis would I rule out their freedom to visit a dermatologist to get advice, or to have non-essential treatment (such as the removal of a mole)? If I accept that people should be free to book restaurants according to their taste, then can I really object to them wanting to pay extra for a chance to pick food of their choice if they have to spend time in hospital? Of course, someone could argue that people exercising their (unequal) resources in this way is 'unfair' but, on that basis and to be consistent, they would need to condemn most discretionary expenditure.

There are some good, positive arguments for encouraging and incentivising collective provision of care – for example, there are advantages in pooling risks and benefits, and the values of community membership and social solidarity entail a concern for ensuring decent provision for the most economically disadvantaged. But it is very difficult to move from these arguments to the conclusion that all private consumption of healthcare should be outlawed. The most that might reasonably be argued (although this would of course be contested by economic liberals) is that people should not be allowed to opt out of collective forms of healthcare financing such as state taxation or social insurance schemes, and that there should be limits to the advantages that people with additional resources are able to buy (that is, that everyone should have a roughly equal chance of benefiting in a timely fashion from a decent package of care provision). Striking a balance between the claims of individual freedom and those of social justice – whether in healthcare or more generally – is a notoriously contentious and divisive issue that I will not pursue further here. But there are other arguments both for limiting and for encouraging freedom to consume health-related goods that deserve consideration.

As mentioned in the last chapter, there is widespread acceptance that people should not be able to buy and sell whatever they want on an unrestricted market. The quality, safety and sale of all medicines, including over-the-counter medicines, is heavily regulated. Similar advertising and safety legislation applies to most products, including health-related products. Also, in the vast majority of cases, people who claim to be 'health practitioners' of various kinds need to register with bodies and agencies that control access to the occupation and specify standards. All of these measures serve to protect consumers' interests in areas where they may lack the expertise to be critical consumers or where they may be in a particular vulnerable state or lacking capacity to make the necessary discriminations themselves. Such regulations and standards also help to underpin collective welfare and public health. However, within these parameters, there is also widespread acceptance that marketplace freedoms are beneficial because, in general, they enable people to make richly informed, sensitive and flexible decisions in ways that reflect their specific circumstances, needs and preferences. To accept this it is not necessary to argue that individuals always know what is best for them. Rather, all one has to accept is (a) that the real value of a product or service is the value it has for the individual(s) it affects (as discussed before, the value of goods is not impersonal and fixed) and (b) that individuals are thus often better placed to judge what they might benefit from than are other people, such that we should err on the side of not taking consumption judgements out of their hands (allowing for exceptions such as capacity questions).

But this same logic can be applied to the use of common or public resources. If, in many instances, we think that individuals are best placed to utilise their personal financial resources in ways that address their own concerns and values, then there seems to be an analogous argument for the suggestion that some pooled or shared resources (that could be devoted to them) should also be 'handed over' to their discretion. Of course there are objections to this suggestion that are worth noting – there are, for example, arguments about the relative efficiency of collective purchasing based upon economies of scale, and there are arguments for having public accountability mechanisms and restrictions in place to stop wasteful expenditure. But there are also, to repeat, arguments in favour of 'handing over' resources. This is a line of reasoning followed, for example, by those who advocate the use of vouchers to encourage both user engagement and market competition in welfare provision – giving people some element of choice over provision and thereby some influence in the marketplace. I will not be reviewing this example here but I do want to consider another application of the same broad idea – the use of 'personal health budgets'.

NHS England began a pilot programme for personal health budgets in 2009, and rolled the policy out further from 2012. Personal health budgets allow the people who get them a great deal of flexibility to spend an allocated budget in ways that match their needs and circumstances. Even though this is a significant departure from the NHS's history, in which patients are not normally given direct access to, or discretion over, the use of NHS resources, it is important to stress at once (especially for those who are strongly committed to collective expenditure) that this scheme is very far from a 'free for all'. It is restricted to comparatively few people who qualify because of complex needs arising out of a long-term condition or disability. The budgets concerned are limited and represent only one component of the monies spent by the NHS on the relevant patients. And, in addition, personal health budgets are not 'free floating' interventions but are embedded in a joint care-planning approach that involves health professionals as well as patients. Access to these budgets is presented by NHS England, for understandable reasons, as one of the personalisation policies it has put in place.

These kinds of personal health budgets – involving the re-allocation of pooled resources to individuals – provide a clear illustration of the health-policy dilemmas arising from personalisation. In particular they illustrate some of the potential tensions between standardised and tailored interventions and the difficulty of drawing boundaries between healthcare goods and other goods. If we take the idea of person-centred healthcare seriously, then we are required to think about the ways in which disease or other ill-health is related to people's broader well-being or quality of life. This means, for example, as is already routine, medical treatments being chosen in a way that reflects people's life-style and concerns; for example, one person might prefer to have a slightly less effective drug that is simple to take, whereas another person may be happy to schedule a complex drug regimen for some small additional benefit. But it also means that attending to 'non-medical' factors may sometimes – in terms of the difference it makes to the experience of living with and coping with ill-health – make an even more significant difference to the impact of ill-health on an individual's quality of life.

For example, an individual with chronic breathing difficulties that are affecting their mobility and causing them to feel socially isolated may benefit in multiple ways from being supported to attend a 'singing for health' choir. Yet, of course, this will not be the best intervention for everyone. People with very similar experiences of ill-health and receiving identical medical treatments will sometimes benefit from very different personal and social interventions. While Danny might be interested and motivated to go to 'singing for health', Harry might respond much better from support to regularly visit his daughter who not only raises his spirits but also motivates and supports him in other activities, including his gentle exercise regime. They have different lives, and different life projects and priorities. The use of personal health budgets can help to facilitate these kinds of interventions and, most relevant for the purposes of this chapter, can allow for the considerable flexibility and responsiveness needed. Personal health budgets are defended by NHS England because they allow for this flexibility and because they allow patients greater control over their lives – something that is both instrumentally and intrinsically important to their well-being.[1]

However, these same factors have made personal health budgets controversial. From time to time they have featured in media stories that call their defensibility into question. For example, in September 2014 the BBC news gave considerable exposure to concerns that had been aired by *Pulse*, a magazine for primary healthcare doctors (General Practitioners or GPs), under the headline 'NHS personal health budgets spent on "patient treats"'.[2] *Pulse* had used the Freedom of Information Act to find out how the money allocated to personal health budgets had been spent in the previous year. On this basis it reported that millions of pounds had been spent and that thousands of this were spent on things that might normally be regarded as treats; examples cited included: new clothes, a sat nav, music and art lessons, a computer game, horse riding, a summer-house, massage and aromatherapy. A British Medical Association (BMA) spokesperson was quoted as saying that the BMA continued to have real reservations about the scheme and 'the inappropriate use of scarce NHS money on non-evidence based therapies'. The deputy chairman of the BMA's General Practitioners' committee, said: 'While individuals may themselves value a massage or summer house, others will understandably start to question why they can't also have such things paid for by the state – and that will just fuel demand.'

The editor of *Pulse* was quoted as saying that his readers had reacted to the story with 'dismay': 'Doctors have to follow the evidence, they have to make sure everything they do is effective. To see in other areas of the NHS money maybe being spent on things that doesn't have such evidence behind it, particularly at a time when the NHS is trying to save lots of money, is hard to swallow.'

The BBC also quoted defenders of the scheme, who argued that the whole idea of 'bespoke' spending was to allow for innovative forms of expenditure rather than what was conventionally or standardly purchased by the NHS, and who underlined the fact that the allocation and spending of budgets was not done without oversight but was done in partnership with health professionals.

The controversy, and the more measured debates, around personal health budgets provide a valuable lens on key aspects of personalisation. They show that attending to individual people's different life circumstances and life projects may require imaginative and unconventional thinking on the part of healthcare providers and, in turn, that this may raise worries about both wasteful expenditure and fairness. But they may also show – whether or not we are ultimately in favour of such a policy – that we should be careful before rushing to judgement about these matters. The BBC, in the same report, provides a case study that illustrates this nicely. It is an example of someone whose family used part of his budget to buy a better TV package with a hard drive that allowed for flexible TV viewing:

> Malcolm Royle's family decided a care home would not be right for him after he developed dementia symptoms in 2005. They used a personal care budget of £46,000 to devise their own care plan, which allowed him to live at home until he died in April. One of the items they bought him was a Sky+ box.
>
> Mr Royle's son, Colin, said: 'It might seem quite an unusual item to purchase with NHS money but it was a great success and the outcomes were terrific.
>
> 'We were able to record all of his favourite television programmes and play them at times of day that suited him as well. We could also fast forward adverts. These caused him a lot of anxiety.'
>
> He added the Sky+ box had ultimately helped to 'stimulate' his father and reduce his anxieties.

From this account – that is, by considering some of the details in a specific case – we can see that judgements about either waste or unfairness are not straightforward. It seems that the 'public' expenditure devoted to this personal budget might otherwise have been used to contribute to the costs of accommodation and care in a residential home. And if we accept that this may not have suited Mr Royle as much as the personalised plan drawn up by his family, then this alternative could have been the really wasteful use of resources. The same applies to the TV box – this is a piece of technology that might provide both comfort and stimulation, in targeted ways, to someone managing the symptoms of dementia. This is not obviously any less of a sensible purchase than any other piece of technology that is available for the health service to buy or supply. Likewise, it is not conspicuously any more unfair that this individual should benefit from NHS money spent by his family on a TV box than that another patient should benefit from dedicated professional expenditure on some other technology. (Some of the worries that arise here are related to the differences between, and the fuzzy boundaries between, clinical and social care, which I will come back to in the next chapter.)

Indeed the case for similar kinds of targeted and flexible public expenditure support for individualised purchasing decisions becomes even stronger if we see them in the context of broader 'social welfare' expenditures and against the backcloth of social and economic inequalities. The broad rationale for social welfare spending (such as on housing, disability benefits, unemployment benefits or in-work benefits for the low-paid) is to provide a humane safety net, or to redistribute wealth and income to support a decent minimum standard of living, for relatively disadvantaged people. In this context – and assuming that we accept these norms (which obviously some might question) – then those who are suffering from long-term conditions or analogous disabilities already have a prima facie case for collective support. If we add in the fact that such conditions can lead to (or be produced by, or simply coincide with) other forms of disadvantage, including financial disadvantage, then this case grows stronger. These kinds of welfare measures can be seen as underpinning solidarity with, basic fairness towards and a measure of independence for members of the community who may not have some of the advantages that many others take for granted (such as the ability to buy and benefit from a TV box.) Of course, in practice, there are notorious problems in working out and applying fair and effective ways of allocating expenditure (for example, having a complex long-term condition does not necessarily coincide with financial hardship), but I am leaving those aside here.

I am not attempting to defend this form of personal health budgets here because this would depend upon a much closer theoretical examination of issues of principle as well as empirical investigation of specific cases. But I am suggesting that the scepticism and hostility about them that is sometimes expressed in the media is overdone. A defence would require consideration of some broader factors – for example, whether their existence, or their significant expansion, could have overall negative effects on the character, and political legitimacy, of organisations like the NHS. It would also include consideration of the 'within programme' fairness just mentioned – for example, is it fair that some sub-set of patients have access to these levels of 'choice' and 'control' and others do not? Both these considerations played a part in the concerns expressed by the editor of *Pulse*, who suggested that the policy 'may give a lot of choice to a small number of patients but actually, overall, it might actually reduce choice'.

Although in many respects using purely private expenditure to 'personalise' health-related consumption is a different matter there are some important commonalities with publicly funded personal health budgets. For example, as discussed above, individual private sector buyers may often need protection from unsafe products, or services that are poor or based upon misleading claims, or at least access to sources of authoritative and trusted guidance on the potential pros and cons of purchasing decisions. These safeguards are loosely analogous to the oversight and partnership elements built into personal health budgets. In addition, such safeguards need to be informed by broader public health and public interest concerns. For some people the latter will include the social justice implications of such 'private' decisions, including their effects on equality of access to healthcare services and experiences. The additional private consumption opportunities afforded by the advance of personalised medicine are no different in this respect, and sceptical attention and safeguards need to be developed with regard to them and underpinned by collective mechanisms and public scrutiny. In short, personalisation – in whatever form – will have costs as well as benefits. And these costs are not simply financial but include the various ways in which the enactment of personalisation policies transforms or inflects the other values and purposes that we would like to see embedded in our health systems.

Personalised care: mixing support with humanity

The discussion of personal health budgets has indicated some of the ways in which personalisation can be thought about as responsiveness to individual biography rather than, or independently of, individual biology. Disease and disability, along with ill-health and the threat of ill-health more generally, cut into people's lives and experiences in different ways. As well as being able to describe underlying anatomical, physiological or biochemical dysfunctions or impairments in relatively detached scientific terms we can, of course, talk about the experiences of ill-health or disability in personal and social terms. This includes not only the ways in which underlying conditions can influence or frame people's life-worlds and create their sense of identity (negatively and/ or positively) but also the ways that the particular social conditions individuals operate within help to produce these experiences and identities, and provide specific constraints on (or opportunities in) their lives.

This is not to deny that there are also very many commonalities between people, such that it is often possible to identify with, and empathise with, other people's sickness and the existential and practical challenges it represents for them. But, of course, an important element of such empathy is not to assume that we can easily or fully identify with what someone else is experiencing or imagine what it is like to be in their specific social circumstances. People's health-related experiences are diverse. It is not just that people may have different symptoms or experience symptoms differently, or that people have different personalities and characters (that is, may differ in temperament and as agents), but also that they have different life histories and social trajectories. This means that the significance and implications of the same 'objective' dysfunction (where this is construed largely in biomedical terms) are potentially very different for different people. If, as a result of an injury, I was advised never to play rugby again it would make no difference to my life; but for someone else this advice could be devastating. If I was advised to seek personal counselling, then I am in a position to afford it, but for someone else this may not only be unattainable (unless funded) but also may seem like a luxury with low priority, given other pressing worries. This is all fairly simple to state even though responding to this diversity is complex.

What matters to people and what people are in a position to do (more or less easily) varies. This is why it is important to plan and deliver care in ways that are responsive to individual peoples' values and lives. Up to a point this is uncontroversial and unproblematic. We should start from the assumption that health policy can encourage and accommodate some degree of personalised care planning. Without it, resources will be used ineffectively because people will not be getting the help and care they need and value. For example, in relation to clinical treatments individuals can be encouraged to share their hopes about how these relate to their life priorities, and they can be supported, within funding and other parameters, to help choose the clinical interventions that they feel suit them and meet their needs best. This broad idea is now a policy orthodoxy. But as we move from the emphasis on 'shared decision-making' – which is often used to refer to one-off, *within* consultation partnership working – towards the full implications of 'support for self-management' or 'individualised care planning' – that is, towards more long-term and open-ended forms of planning around biographical factors – then the potential for controversy grows. These controversies are linked to uncertainties about boundaries – boundaries between professional roles and 'private' lives, and boundaries between health systems and other social systems such as social care systems. We saw some of this in the last section and I cannot cover all the potential sources of controversy here. These controversies are also, in large part, about the extent to which it is practicable, efficient and fair to orient health systems to the lives and priorities of individuals – including when this might be seen as an expression of the common good and when as something that undermines the common good.

One closely related area of contestation that I will not discuss further here because of my emphasis on tailoring healthcare to individuals – and despite its fundamental importance – is worth mentioning because it highlights the potential size of the gulf between biological and biographical tailoring. That is, if we wanted healthcare to be responsive to the values and priorities of individuals there would be no reason to assume that such values would be purely self-regarding. It seems reasonable to assume that individuals will have projects and goals that are centred on other people's well-being (whether, for example, they be friends or family members, peers who are subject to the same services or treatments as themselves or, animated by broader personal commitments to solidarity, whole communities). In this sense being responsive to individuals, or determining what most 'suits' individuals, may take us even further away from the details of their biological constitution and towards their social and civic roles and priorities.

But, sticking to a fairly simple individualist conception of personalising care, it is arguable that some important forms of personalisation are an inherent and taken-for-granted feature of all care planning. When two or more people sit down to undertake the task of care planning a number of things are going on. As well as the process of identifying and differentiating between a range of possibilities and priorities, there is the business of thinking about feasibilities and the distribution of responsibilities – what realistically can be done and whose job is it? In addition, there is the immediate activity of mutual attention, listening and conversation. There is potentially a substantial intrinsic value attached to the processes of recognition and participation that are embedded in care planning. It is important to be conscious of these parallel activities and to see how they can connect personalisation with both 'enablement' and 'empathy'. I will say a little more about each of these linked concerns.

First, let us suppose that – along the lines of the discussion of personal care budgets above – part of the conversation is about the individual having help or support to meet some life goals, for example, to get some new clothes. It is immediately clear that everything depends upon the case and context – what kind of support do they want and why? There will be huge variations in their personal circumstances, existing resources and life projects. If they are unwell or have some other kind of mobility problem then they may simply be looking for interventions that help them to get out of the house and travel around, perhaps including adjustments to their treatments or equipment that are compatible with spending time away from home. If they are looking for some more direct practical or financial help and have very worn clothes and no money to replace them that seems very different than if they have wardrobes full and just like to shop. Of course in all cases there is the question of how far a particular agency should devote human or financial resources to help meet these ends, whether they are construed as needs or wants. But at the very least there seems to be a good reason to listen to people's expressed preferences and to take them seriously in the first instance, to think about how they might be addressed and through what kinds of help from different sources, if only so as to discriminate between those that merit attention and those that (even after consideration) seem trivial, misplaced or even simply selfish.

Personalised care planning thus needs to combine attention to individuals' values and preferences and to the specific conditions of their lives – as currently constituted and in relation to desirable futures – because these conditions create a constellation of constraints and opportunities that shape people's chances of living their lives according to their values and preferences. Practitioners who participate in these processes will also inevitably be 'filtering' these considerations through (a) some conception – depending on their professional and institutional roles – of where they themselves have appropriate expertise and resources and who else they might call upon, and (b) some conception – albeit no doubt one that is contestable – of relative need and priority. Nonetheless, with these necessary complications acknowledged, care planning can, in this sense of helping people towards the lives they want to lead, be aimed at 'enablement'.

Second, as noted above, care planning can in itself be one form of care. There is much that matters in healthcare that is over and above successful outcomes, including 'health' outcomes (Entwistle et al, 2012). The attention and mutuality required by joint planning is one way in which care can be demonstrated. Of course there need not be a clear forward-looking orientation to care. Caring processes can also take a retrospective form, for example, when someone helps to jointly 'take stock' of someone's illness and life experiences and trajectory.

It is arguable that nearly all care, by definition, tends towards something 'personalised' in the sense of individually tailored. Certainly there are 'caring behaviours', sometimes very important ones, that can be enacted with relatively little regard for the specifics of the person who is the target of care. If a busy critical care nurse makes the effort to touch the arm of someone who is undergoing an uncomfortable or frightening procedure this can make a huge difference and, in most respects, it does not matter who the patient is or what, in general, matters to them. This is one aspect of person-centred care – care that is responsive to the suffering of the patient, embodies connection and manifests a humanity that is common if not always commonplace. Many such 'physical' behaviours or acts of caring – especially if routinely repeated – play a crucial role in the contributions that physical and social care can make to well-being and these can easily be under-estimated. But beyond, and often within, this basic or foundational level caring typically requires a degree of engagement with the specific 'standpoint' of the individual concerned.

Mutuality, personal connection and engagement with a subjective standpoint is one dimension of biographical personalisation but it may, under some circumstances at least, seem to fall short of practical caring. To borrow the classic 'Samaritan-type' example – if I am walking down the street and the person beside me falls over, dropping his things on the floor, and hurts his legs in the fall, it might be invaluable if I were to stop and acknowledge how disturbing that experience must be and to show an understanding of his predicament. But it would be odd, and also arguably uncaring, if I did not help to pick his belongings up and check whether he would be OK to go on his way. Indeed he may not only value the practical assistance that I could provide (or call for from someone else) as much as the empathy, but also see it as a concrete affirmation of the empathy. If I am to tailor my response effectively I will need to think in terms of overlapping communicative and causal interventions (or, in Habermas' terms, combine a communicative interest in mutual understanding with an instrumental interest in outcomes). Health and social care professionals, and other carers, are often in a broadly analogous position. That is, they will often not only be in a position to attend to, and connect with, the standpoints and narratives of individuals but also be in a position to do specific things to alter the objective circumstances (and not only the biomedical condition) of those individuals in ways that are of specific benefit to them. The objective changes can vary hugely in scope. If someone is 'gasping for a drink', then, in addition to sympathy, they might be provided with some tea; if someone is living in a damp house, then, in addition, to our genuine concern, they might be directly or indirectly helped to move to accommodation that better suits their needs.

How these two dimensions of biographical personalisation can best be combined, and by whom and when, gives rise to many possible uncertainties and disputes over and above those raised by 'biological personalisation' (or personalised medicine in the restricted sense). Both aspects of biographical personalisation have substantial implications for resources, including human capacity. In addition, they might easily pull in slightly different directions – requiring carers to strike a balance between efforts invested in 'empathy' and 'enablement'. The dilemmas here are very familiar from our personal lives whenever we are faced with friends who face challenges, and our well-intentioned efforts can sometimes be misplaced in either direction.

One of the paradigms that is sometimes cited here, and for good reason, is 'ideal type' care of the dying. Although saying so risks sounding trite, when someone dies, or is coming to the end of their life, we are reminded of what is important and how people 'deserve' to be treated. Such care includes the sheer presence of other persons who – assuming they are suitable persons and 'present' in the right way – can diminish the existential threat of isolation. But it can also include much more textured and 'detailed' kinds of mutuality – listening to, and talking about, people's fears and hopes; engaging with immediate and prosaic concerns alongside longer-term reflections and stories; helping someone be 'heard' – whether that means being subject to cries of anguish, attending to people's narratives and 'search for meaning' (Frankl, 2004) or actively supporting efforts to find forms of order. Of course 'presence' and sense making will usually be accompanied by other kinds of 'tailored' interventions, including the management of physical pain and the control of disease symptoms and also help with personal belongings and plans, access to friends and family, and adjustments to life circumstances.

This is also a paradigm example of where some neat technical intervention (however tailored) will be radically insufficient. It is why healthcare has to be seen in the light of what some authors call a 'service logic' and not just a 'product logic' (Osborne, Radnor and Nasi, 2013; Batalden et al, 2015). On this account we need to distinguish between the policy, management and practice logics that apply to two different kinds of 'goods' – products and services. A service is distinguished from a product in three key respects: because it consists in significant part of 'intangible' elements (as well as concrete elements); because the activities of the production and consumption of the goods in question happen at the same time and place (are inseparable from one another); and because the goods in question are co-produced through the interaction between services and service users. This account of a practice logic that is appropriate for services reinforces my argument about the nature of personalised care. Specifically, it indicates that personalisation cannot be achieved by the concrete elements of health-related goods alone – even when this includes specifically tailored biotechnology or the provision or consumption of other individually chosen or fitted products – but only by active engagement with the person. But it is worth underlining that key authors in this area such as Osborne and Radnor argue that this insight about the distinctive nature of a service logic extends far beyond discussions of personalisation and has relevance across much of public service. The suggestion is not that product logics are irrelevant – there are situations where service logics have less relevance and product logics, underpinned by the kinds of bureaucratic and standardising rationales discussed in the last chapter, are more appropriate. In these cases biographical engagement is less called for, or at least less central. This account of service logic suggests that the notion of personalisation embodied in what I have called personalised care is valuable not because it illuminates something unique or special but because it highlights a widespread feature of much of healthcare properly understood.

I am suggesting that the aspiration to care is neither conceptually nor practically meaningful unless it is responsive to people as individuals. Caring in this sense is not just being responsive to biography but is, in part, 'doing' biography – helping people to make sense of their lives and, at the same time, participating with them in those lives. And, in this sense, it is impossible to have 'non-personalised' care. To repeat, this conception of care has relevance across all of healthcare. The threats to coping and identity, the threat of isolation and the drive to make sense of our experiences are general features of human life and the ever-present possibility of suffering it entails. If health systems are to be configured to support care and not just health this has very big implications for health policy. It requires us to reconceptualise 'human resources' and – if we are to underpin practice logics for services and not just products – to re-examine the focus and underlying models of both professionalism and policy making.

Obviously I am not arguing that everyone in healthcare roles should be continuously engaged in open-ended 'biographical work'. There would arguably be no end to such work. Paying attention to someone's biography is an indefinitely large task. There are many healthcare contexts and interventions in which it is not central to what is needed, and there are comparatively few circumstances in which it falls to a health professional or other non-family carer to take on this task in more than modest ways. But I would argue that this kind of work has general relevance, is often a very central element of decent care and should always be 'close to hand' in healthcare institutions. To neglect it in healthcare planning might be seen as the equivalent of neglecting the supply of oxygen or blood to the system. Furthermore, in very many instances – such as helping people to manage long-term conditions – personalised care (in the sense of biographical working) is simply a necessary condition of doing an adequate job.

Conclusion

As with both 'choice' and 'holism', the subjects of the previous two chapters, personalisation is *both* an important idea to have in a policy-reforming toolkit *and* an idea that requires a good deal of unpacking and some measure of caution. I have concluded the chapter by reflecting on the challenges of combining two different facets of personalised care or 'biographical working'; but the main issue I wanted to highlight in this chapter is the gap between, and challenge of combining, biological and biographical tailoring, or personalised medicine and personalised care. If anything, I have underplayed the size of the potential gap here. Services that were responsive to what matters to individuals would likely not be solely tailored around those individuals but would be designed to serve collective ends and common goods – because people are embedded in and value these things. However – even just sticking with individually tailored healthcare – what I would like to underline, in a nutshell, is that personalised medicine needs to be firmly anchored in personalised care. Some of the key risks associated with personalised medicine – including the risks that it might be applied wastefully or unfairly – are exacerbated if it is not nested within personalised care.

Unless medical interventions are geared towards the things that matter to patients they will not only be ineffective but might also be judged to be harmful or even, when insufficient care is taken to respect autonomy, simply wrong. However well designed and targeted a biological intervention, or however well customised or conducted a social intervention, these things will not be 'tailored' in the critical sense unless they are part of personalised care. This proposition is easy to defend in principle, but there are reasons to worry that it may be difficult to comply with in practice. In part this is because it is not always straightforward to identify what personalised care demands – it requires sustained attention to, and engagement with, what matters to individuals, including, for example, attention to what might reasonably be expected to come to matter to them. This is not an exact science and leaves room for well-intentioned error at the margins. But it is also because even when we get these judgements right they are not the only things that determine what happens in practice. As discussed at length in Chapter Two, the power of biomedical discourses and norms to shape practice is considerable and this means that there is always a danger that what happens is overly driven by biomedical possibilities and norms in ways that risk 'floating free' of what personalised care would demand. Drivers of practices that are not anchored in personalised care can, for example, arise from the powerful impetus of markets that 'sell' personalised medicine. And even if such 'selling' were to be responsible and hit the target the danger is that, overall, the market rationale for personalisation will, in practice, eclipse the social justice rationale (see Mladenov et al, 2015). In other words the danger is that personalisation may be constructed so narrowly that increasingly refined packages of treatment will be available to a few people but that many others, who face substantial structural disadvantages with regard to the conditions that shape their health experiences, are bypassed.

Notes

[1]   See www.england.nhs.uk/healthbudgets/ for this account and examples.
[2]   www.bbc.co.uk/news/health-34110964.

SIX

The challenge of integration

This book is organised around the argument that a central challenge for health policy making and practice is 'holding things together' – that is, finding ways of providing, supporting or enacting different kinds of goods at the same time. The last three chapters give an indication of some of the tensions that are embedded in discourses of 'person centred' healthcare – not just tensions between currents that extend the biomedical model and those that seek to erode or work outside it, but also tensions that arise both within and across different facets of person-centred thinking. These worries about tensions can be translated into a set of policy challenges: How can we best combine (forms of) choice with (forms of) care? (More broadly how can we harness people's agency but in ways that do not indiscriminately 'off-load' responsibility and exacerbate inequalities?) How can we combine proper attention to the needs and interests of populations with those of individuals; and how can we design and operate care systems that do both? When attending to individuals, how far can we embed biological tailoring within biographical tailoring? And how, more generally, can we work with both causal and communicative ways of relating to persons? This list is not meant to be exhaustive but merely to represent the tensions featured in the last few chapters and to indicate the kinds of challenges I have in mind in this chapter.

This chapter focuses on the challenge of combining or integrating goods. Although it is not typically expressed in such abstract or generic terms this is a challenge that is well recognised in health-policy contexts and I will begin by discussing some of the familiar ways in which it is already manifest and managed. This will illustrate some of the structural, logistical and practical hurdles we need to overcome in order to plan services that address diverse concerns in a way that is broadly coordinated. Following that I will argue that running through and underlying these familiar examples there are more fundamental challenges facing integration that need to be acknowledged and addressed. Indeed I will argue that the business of integration symbolises both the importance and the difficulties attached to the philosophical transition that forms the theme of this book.

My overall interest is in endorsing the value of integration, but in order to do that it is necessary to distinguish between different conceptions of, elements of and purposes served by integration. Specifically I will argue that we need to be suspicious of a search for a 'policy alchemy' through which all relevant goods can be magically combined together without loss. At least we need to be conscious that the way integration is valued by services may not capture all the ways in which integration might be valued by service users and others. I want to suggest that thinking about integration is one way of attending to shifts in the locus of agency in health policy and to how the philosophical transition I am reviewing requires us to consider healthcare goods and action from multiple standpoints. There is also an important 'material' element to the question of combination. Ideas about good care cannot simply be combined and held together in some weightless and frictionless realm of thought. So although my emphasis, here as elsewhere, is on the underlying models or 'logics' involved in healthcare transitions I will also pay some attention to the socio-material dimension of integration within health systems.

Divisions and boundaries

It is not difficult to find the broad idea of 'integration' in policy discourses. It is, for example, implicit in the very widespread and prominent discourses around 'partnership' or 'collaboration' (and similar notions) that indicate the coming together of people or agencies that might otherwise be on different trajectories. Words like 'partnership' imply a coming together that is constructive, successful and perhaps even harmonious. (I will say something about the frictions and other 'problems' of partnership working later.) Partners – as in the case of the individual professional–patient partnerships discussed in Chapter Three – may have different concerns, priorities and forms of expertise, but the ideal is that these can effectively be brought together through collaborative efforts. The different things that matter to, and can be achieved by, different people can thereby be integrated into the best possible shared outcome or set of goods. Something closely analogous is sought, or at least suggested, by policies directed at the level of agencies or sectors, through the development of inter-professional, multi-agency or cross-sectoral partnership working.

In order to approach the integration agenda it is worth acknowledging the 'problem' that gives rise to it. The agenda is closely bound up with divisions and boundaries that are both necessary and (equally necessarily) a source of difficulties. The way in which health systems seek to provide diverse goods is through a division of labour that structures both services and roles. This is unavoidable. Without this division of labour everyone would be aiming to do everything, and this is an idea that is not merely impractical but borders on being unintelligible. Yet the necessary division of labour inevitably and notoriously creates problems – how can contributions be coordinated; how will people and information move between services; will some needs fall through the cracks; how can we minimise duplications and inefficiencies; and so on? Such problems are unavoidable because, although services and roles have to be separated out, people's well-being needs cannot be tidily separated out into components but are always clustered together in people's lives.

Perhaps the central device through which health policy addresses and manages this tension – between differentiated provision and consolidated needs – is by supporting both specialism and generalism. This is, of course, a recognised feature of the division of labour in healthcare. In both medicine and nursing, for example, some services and professional roles are constructed as more specialist and some as more generalist. Interventions that require very particular expertise, equipment and institutional arrangements can be assigned to specialist staff or units, while other staff or units can contribute to, and maintain an overview of, a patient's overall care – something that is very roughly reflected in a number of important structural arrangements in health services, including the broad distinction between primary and secondary provision. Primary care, as well as being more generalist is, for analogous reasons, more community based – closer to people's ordinary social lives and the broader networks of social relations and services they are embedded in; whereas secondary care is, as the name implies, typically a further 'step away' from normal life, often in 'separated' spaces.

The challenges and responsibilities of coordination – taking an overview of needs, signposting and supporting people through multiple agencies and keeping in mind people's overall well-being – tend to be associated with generalist services, and often with primary care providers. But, of course, even within specialist roles and practices there is a need to combine the more specific and the general aspects of healthcare. Indeed this distinction is relevant at all levels of health policy, planning and action. Fundamentally this is because there are more specific and general features of health and well-being: someone with a broken leg needs their leg tending to but also may need help with negotiating their everyday life and maintaining their personal and social equilibrium.

Anyone who has an interest in health has to be ready to focus both on things that are health specific (and condition specific) in the narrowest sense and on aspects of general well-being, and to give some thought to how the specific and the general concerns and purposes intersect and what forms of joint working are required to address them both. This makes life difficult. If we could draw neat boundaries around all health-related activities such that they each had circumscribed purposes and effects, and did not interact with one another, this would enable some significant simplifications. Although there would still be need for social coordination and for working across boundaries, the principal concern would be trying to line up the necessary 'intervention elements' in the optimum order. Something akin to this is possible in specific and local cases – for example, if a doctor asks someone to go down the corridor to get a blood test and an X-ray and to come back a couple of hours later. But most cases, even sticking within single healthcare institutions, are not this simple and, without much more careful coordination, raise risks for patients – caused by multiple points of 'service access' that produce barriers and delays, or by service effects undermining rather than supporting one another. These complications are multiplied further when we come to consider the very many ways in which health interventions have implications for personal well-being more broadly.

Under some circumstances being 'lifted out' of our normal lives and environments and placed under close scrutiny in a dedicated setting may be exactly what is needed. But even on these occasions there is a need for good service coordination within and across settings – for example, a period of monitoring and follow-up after hospitalisation, which will rest in part on primary care doctors and nurses, or on involved and informed lay carers or self-management. Similar forms of coordination are routinely needed for the very many people who have long-term health conditions and find themselves having to manage their conditions with help from a range of primary and secondary healthcare services or from voluntary organisations, peers and peer groups. Even more obviously, those people who have to live with multiple conditions and related complications – an ever-increasing number of people as populations age – are not always well served by services and institutional spaces designed around single conditions, but positively require more holistic and responsive environments. In all cases the spheres of clinical care and of 'normal life' in people's homes and communities need to be effectively joined up.

This is what people typically have in mind when they call for more 'integrated' forms of care; and it is why the aspiration to better integrate healthcare has grown and become a prominent policy issue. Furthermore, given the importance of linking clinical experiences and social experiences and of better connecting care with everyday life, the aspiration extends beyond healthcare in a narrow sense and often includes coordination across health and social care. The term 'integrated care' is frequently used in this context, but it would be a mistake to suppose that there was some clear, agreed and singular meaning to the term. It is used with a variety of emphases and connotations. Its force can be best understood, at a foundational level, as being the opposite of 'un-integrated', 'dis-integrated' or 'fragmented' care provision, in just the same way that 'person-centred' care is often invoked as a way of signalling a contrast to narrowly framed biomedical models of care.

A specific policy challenge that has brought some of these boundary-crossing issues to a head, and to public prominence, is the care of frail elderly patients who frequently end up in hospital when they could, in many cases, be 'better' cared for outside hospital, that is, in their own homes, with relatives or in community nursing homes. 'Better' here refers to a variety of things – including that their clinical needs (which may be relatively minor) could be adequately met, but with their 'social needs' being more fully addressed; that they could be in environments that they would prefer to be in and that they would experience as more 'normal' and more compatible with their life histories and identities, with care provided by people – unpaid or paid – who are in a position to be more responsive to them, and that this could often be at less overall cost. Such people are sometimes referred to, in a phrase many find distasteful, not least because of its victim-blaming connotations, as 'bed blockers' – meaning that they are indirectly preventing the full utilisation of scarce hospital beds with serious 'knock-on effects' to hospitals' responsiveness and efficiency.

This is a problem that may seem to have a relatively straightforward solution on paper, but that is much more demanding in reality. The hospital beds and associated staffing being utilised are, by definition, in place, whereas the provision of suitable forms of care in the community may not be, and cannot be simply brought into existence by a magic wand. That is to say, even if the necessary financial resources could be directly lifted out of hospital budgets to compensate relatives who might have to work fewer hours, or to extend the pool of paid carers in the community, then the practicalities of putting suitably flexible, accountable and high-quality community systems and provision in place are quite daunting. Nor is 'community provision' itself cohesive – there are many minor and some major divisions here too, such as those between physical and mental health services, professional and voluntary sectors, state-organised and private sector providers, health and social care agencies and so on. But, of course, financial resources cannot, in any case, be moved that easily. There are often different streams of funding and patterns of payment for different sectors and services. In the UK, for example, people expect the normal care provided to them by NHS hospitals to be free at the point of delivery, but many people would be expected to pay something towards the social care they receive in their homes. Under these circumstances this means that hospital managers and professionals who are aiming to move people across the boundary between hospital and social care are often, in effect, generating financial costs for these people. This may well be as it should be but it is indicative of the complications entailed by care coordination. Although the need and scope for policy and service coordination is very much more extensive than this single example, it is a useful example for indicating both the rationale for, and problems of, integration.

The integration agenda has attained a very high policy profile because of conspicuous service difficulties and shortcomings, such as the example just discussed, but these are only surface manifestations of more pervasive problems and underlying tendencies and tensions. The problems are, in large measure, those that derive from the growing 'mismatch', discussed at the start of Chapter Two, between the historical evolution of services and the changed needs, priorities, expectations and perspectives of service users.

Sam and Esther

In relation to the idea of 'integration' – as in other reforming discourses already discussed – we are often encouraged to invert conventional thinking about system planning. If, instead of starting with the day-to-day challenges of running services, we start from the experience of individuals, or groups experiencing similar risks or burdens, we can ask what patterns of provision and support will make their lives go better, and how we can minimise 'gaps' or 'clashes' in such provision. A device that is used to dramatise, 'humanise' and sensitise policy makers and professionals to the issues in this area is to focus on some hypothetical individuals. How do things look from their point of view? This section title refers to two such individuals.

Sam is a character who appears in a King's Fund animation designed to show the need and potential for integrated care.[1]

Sam is 87 and has emphysema, type 2 diabetes and arthritis; he has lost his wife and is lonely and often depressed. There are times when he cannot manage on his own and calls for help and ends up going in an ambulance to the Emergency

Department, which sometimes leads to him being admitted onto a ward. Although he eventually ends up getting valuable attention he gets frustrated because he is constantly having to explain his various conditions and concerns to lots of different health professionals. In addition, his return home is often delayed because he has to wait until he can be assessed by the relevant social services. Thus he spends a good deal of unnecessary time in hospital, which is very unsatisfactory for him and inefficient for the health service. Even when he gets home the absence of coordination between his GP (primary care doctor) and social services means he doesn't get the support he needs to manage, and so the cycle starts again. As a result of going around in this circle, he is admitted into a care home.

Sam exemplifies the kind of case discussed above. The animation goes on to explain how things might be different and, in particular, how Sam might be better supported at home to enable him to enjoy a better quality of life, more effective care and support and greater independence. This has the effect of making the question of a care home – as and when that becomes relevant – more of a meaningful choice rather than a practical necessity.

Kathy, a district nurse, is given overall responsibility for coordinating Sam's care. Kathy meets with Sam, his primary care doctor and his social worker and Sam explains his needs and preferences, including his preference to manage with his conditions at home. They collectively design a shared care plan. Kathy routinely visits Sam at home to help him with the management of his emphysema and diabetes and also gives him a secure framework and a single person to relate to. If he has a crisis he calls Kathy and not an ambulance. The result is much less frequent visits to the hospital, and also much quicker discharges because of the care plan infrastructure that Kathy keeps in place. In the scenario envisaged here Sam's health and social care is funded through a pooled budget to allow for more holistic and responsive decisions about spending and priorities. He is provided with what he needs to maintain his life at home (for example, a seat in the shower, an oxygen cylinder and a medication dispenser). Equally important, Kathy also helps sets up some social activities as part of a response to Sam's loneliness.

The integration illustrated here – embodied in Kathy and the shared care plan – addresses the fragmentation of services but, most importantly, helps to repair the fragmentation experienced by Sam. The King's Fund stresses, in the presentation of its animation, that this model is not idealistic or unrealistic because something like it already applies in some places. But the challenge it is setting out is how to make this model of thinking and action both more widespread and more taken for granted.

The value of such concrete examples of person–centred thinking is not just that they powerfully illuminate the shortcomings of systems and can suggest alternative possibilities – which is pedagogically valuable for fuelling the emotional and practical imaginations of system actors – but that they, even more valuably, can be harnessed to directly bring about and constitute real–world system change. Such is the case with 'Esther'.

The 'Esther Project Network' originated in one of the areas of Jönköping County, Sweden but has since spread to other areas of Sweden and internationally. 'Esther' is a fictional character invented by a group of providers and health professionals and used to motivate and provide focus for system change in relation to care coordination and more generally. In the first instance Esther was sketched out in fairly specific terms – like Sam – but over time this construction has been relaxed so that the name 'Esther' can also be used a place marker for any potential individual in need of integrated care.

The sketch of the original Esther was as 'a gray-haired, ailing but competent elderly Swedish woman with a chronic condition and occasional acute needs'. This story was elaborated more specifically, including her increasing difficulty with breathing, the oedema in her legs that means she cannot sleep lying down and other mobility problems that make it difficult to manage access to her third-floor apartment. Like's Sam's story, this story goes on to demonstrate some dysfunctional relationships with services that include Esther's having to wait excessively while being passed from agency to agency, professional to professional, in ineffective ways.[2] By working through the situation from Esther's point of view the Esther strategy and project management teams: (a) developed a set of objectives that, in addition to support and security for Esther, included strengthening working relationships across the various agencies, more sharing of information and approaches to documentation, improved capability and quality, and better recording and communication of resulting improvements; (b) translated these objectives into a set of practical system-improvement projects, all of which were organised around and constantly sustained by asking 'What is best for Esther?'

The focus and motivation provided by the Esther project has brought about changes in relationships between patients and professionals, as well as changes in professional relationships and in professional and system norms and expectations. At a structural level the main shift has been to reduce the extent to which the different care agencies and practitioners work independently according to their own agendas. This, for example, has included the development of closer team links and referral relationships between primary care providers and specialists in acute care, which significantly reduce waiting times and rates of hospital admissions, and thereby release resources for further improvements.

The measurable 'gains' in these important system indicators have no doubt contributed to the recognition and the spread of the Esther network. However, this success is also dependent on, and manifest in, a substantial educational and cultural change process that encompasses all parties. This includes, for example, an enhancement of 'patient education' by nurses and other care providers offering more hands-on guidance to support self-management, as well as education for everyone else, including for system leaders, about the need for more integrated approaches to care. The emphasis on the potential importance of self-management reminds us that people such as Sam and Esther should not be thought of as 'passive' beneficiaries of care – they will be looking after themselves already and, in many cases may also be acting as carers for others or making broader contributions to their communities. (Arguably, the biggest division of labour that needs attention is that between official and unofficial forms of care and social action.)

Most substantially, the Esther network has involved an extensive education and training system for networks of providers – who have been challenged, supported and collectively harnessed to 're-think' their assumptions and approaches to providing care. This initiative has included the development of a network of Esther 'coaches', recruited from providers and practitioners who work on the front line with 'Esther' (their own 'Esthers'), and trained to be system coaches, that is, to work across boundaries. In addition, these coaches and other 'change agents' work in partnership with fully involved senior citizens who both complement and critically question the perspectives being shared and developed through coaching sessions. The teams work to advance the understanding and practice of service integration from the 'bottom up'; always encouraging practitioners to think about how to identify and execute Esther's priorities and to use this powerful human lens, and the mutual support of the Network, as a driver of service improvement (Vackerberg et al, 2016).

Realigning relationships: gluing and ungluing connections

Greater coordination of health and social care activities – such as exemplified in the previous section – symbolises the concerns of this book. It can be seen as a consequence of, and one important policy manifestation of, the philosophical transition that I have argued is in process: the realignment of relations between clinical and social spheres, including the closing of distances between 'special' clinical agendas and spaces (physical and cultural) and other social agendas and spaces. Recent policy calls for the greater integration of health and social care reflect both the diffusion of clinical activity across social space and the need for health-system actors, including health professionals, to both respond to and depend upon other social actors.

These realignments in relationships can, as indicated in earlier chapters, be explained partly by the rise in salience of long-term conditions, that is, a world in which many more people are living with and needing – and sometimes actively choosing – to take responsibility for (multiple) chronic conditions often into old age. Hence the relevance of case studies such as those of Sam and Esther. However, the rise in the prevalence and salience in 'physical' long-term conditions (such as diabetes, heart disease and so on) has – as I have noted before –only served to highlight, and raise the profile of, ways of thinking that were already recognised as of crucial importance in many other areas such as social care, mental health promotion, support for people with learning disabilities and, indeed, for people living with disabilities more generally. Namely, it highlights the way people's well-being concerns can often be seen as things that pervade (and sometimes frame) their experience and need to be responded to holistically and in the context of their ongoing lives, personal identities and social relationships. Furthermore, the 'gestalt switch' that is stimulated by, and follows from, thinking about healthcare in ways that are 'fit for' long-term conditions is reinforced by many other aspects of contemporary social change and has relevance across all of healthcare. For example, people increasingly expect to be able to steer their own way through their own lives, and are less prepared for a role of simple 'compliance'. Likewise, hospitalisation for treatment is much rarer and shorter term – and even if this trend is substantially driven by economic considerations it is also compatible with positive philosophies of rehabilitation, self-care, peer support and community action. In a nutshell, people occupy the unequivocal identity of 'patients' less often, and when they do think of themselves as patients this is often a smaller proportion of their self-identity than it once was.

Many have thus come to believe, for good reasons, that the organising models for healthcare need to be transformed. The historically dominant biomedical model has, understandably, tended towards high levels of investment, specialisation and institutional autonomy within multiple divisions of secondary care. Coordination of care is seen to require more investment in primary care and community settings –

where most people spend most of their time and which form the natural place for bringing together groups of people, multiple disease-management activities and health and social agendas more broadly. But greater integration equally depends upon thought, planning and investment in coordination across the whole system. A lot of current reform initiatives are informed by ideas parallel to the Esther Network, that is, can be seen as being about trying to erode the fragmentation within and across health and social care. This can happen, for example, by literally bringing combinations of services together in the same site – producing less physical and cultural distance both between different providers and between providers and users, including embedding some primary care services in secondary settings and vice versa, and providing access to a range of social spaces, welfare and 'holistic services' close to clinical ones.[3] More broadly it entails: blurring the boundaries between sectors; creating roles that are designed to move across boundaries or to help patients and families themselves to navigate landscapes of care and support; conceiving, commissioning and providing packages of care or 'pathways' for individuals or groups of patients that transcend service boundaries; sharing channels of communication or opening up access to information – including information shared with or held by patients. Lying behind all of these things is the recognition that services will tend to develop processes and priorities that reflect their own needs rather than the needs of patients or populations and that, as a corrective to this, care planning should constantly be brought back to the question of what is needed and valued by service users.

The Esther example shows that these forms of rethinking and re-organising are possible, but also that they require considerable effort and entail a great deal more than bringing services together. They also generate both opportunities and complications. Integration of care requires concerted investments of thought, time and resource and the mobilisation of many people. Success can depend upon introducing new roles and bringing different actors into play, including mobilising, and taking seriously, 'lay expertise' and the agency of local actors and communities – shifting not only the centre of attention but also the locus of activity and control in both care provision and policy formation. This degree of difficulty and effort is, of course, why successful reforms, including service realignments, are often small scale and local (or patchy), and not as widespread or sustainable as reforming policy architects would like to see.

But projects that aim for further integration also represent a crucial learning opportunity for health system actors – they provide a chance to work with and attend to the orientations and dispositions of the diverse contributors to lay care and formalised social care, who are used to working in the midst of people's lives. For example, social care system leaders and practitioners – lay or professional – can act as resources for understanding the potential for (and the problems in) doing 'biographical' work in partnership with people individually and collectively – trying to underpin meaningful 'close up' support in a way that has a focus (deploying appropriate expertise) but also responds to people's complexities, preferences and so on. Of course this is not meant to imply that social care workers have solved the relevant set of problems here. It is, rather, that they have considerable familiarity with and experience of 'balancing acts' that are becoming ever more salient for healthcare workers – attempting to balance and (to some degree) 'integrate' professional and personal agendas, and to work 'with' and not only 'for' individuals and communities. In the next section I will explore some of the tensions inherent in the integration agenda in more depth; but to conclude this one I can begin to indicate some of the risks and complications of this agenda.

In a comparatively early discussion paper on the 'meaning, logic and implications' of integrated care Kodner and Spreeuwenberg (2002) underline the person-centred value of integration and also point to its potential for reducing wasted expenditure and contributing to cost-effectiveness. They describe integration as the 'glue' that is needed to hold together the elements of complex health and social care systems. The implication is that without glue such elements may, as we have already seen, be disconnected or constantly splintering. Kodner and Spreeuwenberg also outline what they describe as a 'continuum of strategies' that might serve to foster better integration. In other words, they make suggestions about the 'glue' that might be needed. The broad strategies and some of the specific considerations they consider include:

- funding – for example, seeing how budgets might be pooled and how commissioning can be combined;
- administration – for example, planning across sectors; reviewing patterns of decentralisation and consolidation, joining up needs-assessment processes;
- organisation – for example, exploring co-location, improving discharge and transfer processes, joint management of services, mergers, alliances or networks;
- service delivery – for example, integrated information systems; inter-disciplinary teamwork and case management, joint training;

- clinical care – e.g. a common language, shared clinical records, joint care planning, common decision-support tools. (from Kodner and Spreeuwenberg, 2002)

This list of possibilities – which chimes with the above examples, is still recognisable as relevant 15 years later, and roughly entails reforming all of the facets of healthcare – usefully indicates the breadth and depth of practical change needed to enhance integration. Each of the factors indicated – and these could be unpacked, elaborated and augmented at much greater length – relate to things that are not easy to change. This, in large measure, is because of the sheer inertia that attaches to all social systems (previously discussed in relation to the idea of 'path dependency'). That is, even if there was no ambiguity about the weaknesses of current configurations of provision or the relative strengths of reformed configurations, reconfiguration is always hard work. However, there is always also likely to be active resistance to such reconfiguration and this resistance will typically include sincere, and more or less valid, arguments about the merits of the unreformed configurations and the risks posed by change.

The complications can be illustrated through analogy with our ordinary lives. We each have a network of people to whom we might turn for help – perhaps our parents, partners, siblings, nearby and long-distance friends, colleagues, neighbours and so on. Although it is very unlikely that we think in terms of a 'division of labour', we will tend to look to different individuals for different kinds of things, and to do so in parallel and only partly overlapping ways. For the most part the actions of our personal network are not orchestrated. But if someone were to try to achieve this orchestration for a specific reason this could prove difficult. It would not just be an administrative and communication challenge. We might also worry about conflicts arising between individuals or groups who do not normally mix. We may not necessarily want people to share what they know about us with others. We could be concerned that the coordination of efforts might unravel through inadequate levels of organisation, or through 'too much' organisation – that several people would take it upon themselves to be organisers and that the broth would be spoiled by too many cooks. The same complications that apply to coordination between people also apply to the need to orchestrate material resources – 'spaces' and equipment and so on. There are advantages, as well as disadvantages, in things being separated off from one another and 'owned' and controlled by different agents. A lack of coordination between agents is likely to cause problems, but a very heavy emphasis on coordination will likely just cause different problems.

In other words there is already 'glue' in place, and it serves a purpose. Existing social arrangements are inherently 'sticky' – institutions and services, like the buildings that house them, are held together by links that are typically more substantial and stronger than the links between different institutions and services. Analogous things can be said about the people who make up institutions and services – they will often have shared trajectories and common loyalties that lead to strong bonds that are not always easily replicated in newer and more diffuse relationships. These bonds might be, but need not be, those that exist between professional or managerial 'tribes' or groups – they might well include loyalties within inter-professional teams or long-standing networks. Historically embedded forms of organisation and relationships – even if the rationale that gave rise to them is no longer as credible as it once was – are likely to adhere together. But it would be a mistake to see this existing glue simply in terms of inertia or conservatism. In many cases existing institutional, team or network loyalties play an important role. They serve particular functions, maintain cohesiveness, underpin motivations and efficiencies, and they can provide solace when efforts seem unpromising or unrewarded. Integration of care thus means applying new types of glue while recognising the value of existing types of glue and not inadvertently breaking things up that have value. In the case of the greater integration of health and social care, for example, we need to be conscious of the possible advantages of the prior division of labour, and of service and role separation, as well as of those of integration.

Integration unpacked

In the remainder of this chapter I want to raise some concerns about the ideal of integration. This is partly just following through the notion that integration has risks and costs as well as benefits. But I also want to underline the fact that there are philosophical as well as practical constraints facing integration, and that there are different conceptions of integration that might provide different kinds of guide to the coordination challenges that health policy faces. The practical constraints on integration include the financial, organisational, logistical and psychological 'costs' and risks of change – the burdens of, and brakes on, reconfiguration. The philosophical constraints arise because: first, integration has different elements and purposes – it is not just about increasing the practical links between, and efficiencies across, services but about changes in personal and social identities and relationships; and second, in so far as it is about services or professionals working together it is important to remember these are often doing very different things, operate according to different 'logics' and cannot necessarily be combined without conflict. I will begin by developing this second point, but gradually say more about the first and broader point.

The recognition that different professional groups occupy different positions in social and ideological space – that they are acting from different perspectives and in contexts where different things are salient – can be generalised to the many other relevant actors, including lay actors. This should make us further question any 'unifying' or 'totalising' implications that might be associated with the notion of integration. We typically, and sensibly, think about successful integration as about some degree of coordination across services rather than as a comprehensive amalgamation of services, that is, we recognise the distinctive functions of different services and the value of separation between these functions. The importance of maintaining some degree of separation and 'untidiness' can be illustrated by considering two of the types of 'glue' highlighted by Kodnor and Spreeuwenberg – a common approach to information sharing and a common professional framework.

A little reflection will indicate that it is unclear how far common or shared frameworks – either for information or for 'professionalism' – are practicable or a good thing. People who are doing different jobs need to access different kinds of information in different ways. This is obvious if we take sharply contrasting cases. Someone who is monitoring a patient's response to an evolving drug regime will ideally want access to a range of clinical measures. Someone who is helping to support the same person's access to, or participation in, local voluntary agencies will need very different data not only about local services but about the person's way of life and preferences. The former will rightly wish to place a few quantitative measures centre stage, the latter will need to focus on a more diffuse set of data, including some relatively open-ended 'softer' and perhaps narrative-based data. Of course it is technically possible that much of this data might be recorded in, or uploaded into, one place – and there may well be significant advantages in this. However, which information is used, how it is used and how regarded as salient will vary from agent to agent. The importance of this divergence becomes stark if we move away from thinking of the data base as simply a giant storage book and towards thinking of it as an information technology tool or as part of an 'intelligent learning system'. For whom would the tool be programmed – what kinds of reminders or alerts would it issue, what progress would it monitor, what would appear on the dashboard screen and what would be contained in folders at lower levels? Different services and agents would certainly produce different specifications in this regard. This corresponds with the fact that different professions are – to note something that is true by definition but also substantively important – designed to be different from one another. The pluralism provided by different agencies and professional roles and perspectives represents something of considerable importance. The idea of a 'common professional framework' might make sense if it is understood as a very broad 'common space' in which professionals can come together, compare notes and pursue greater coordination of activities (as illustrated above), but it makes little sense to imagine some merging of perspectives into a generic professionalism.

This can be illustrated by imagining that some new practitioner role is developed to provide home care and support to individuals such as Sam or Esther. What should such a person do? The doctor who is measuring the effects of a new drug regime might, for example, like them to check that they are adhering to the medicines regime and to record some clinical readings. The social worker who is trying to help maintain a network of social opportunities and activities might like them to engage in conversation to explore options and preferences, or to escort individuals to a new local group on a trial basis. Other professional and lay carers – the occupational therapy service, the memory clinic, the neighbours who help with the laundry and so on – will have their own ideas as to aspects of their caring agendas that could be usefully followed up. In addition, and not least, the individual being supported may themselves have lots of other ideas about what they would welcome – help with shopping, or with the new television that seems harder to operate than the previous one, or with a Skype call to important but distant relatives, or perhaps discussion of current affairs and politics (or some other long-standing passion).

Of course the person appointed might do very many of these things. It would certainly be good to have someone whose role was fairly flexible and responsive, and someone who was ready to take an overview both of which things were or were not being done and of what other formal or informal help was available to refer to or call upon. This kind of flexible role is key to the aspiration for integrated care and undoubtedly to be welcomed. However, in reality such a role could not and would not be completely open ended. There would be some job description and associated 'person specification', there would be some defined lines of reporting and accountability; there might even be some quite prescriptive objectives or 'targets' that had to be recorded and met in order for funding to be justified or sustained. Relative open-endedness is not the same as shapelessness and, of course, in some respects it is a very good thing that everyone – certainly including the individual at the centre – has a reasonably clear understanding of what the role is and is not, and of what might count as relative 'success' in the role (and what falls outside the remit and is thus not relevant to role success, although it may be important in other respects). In other words, the 'division of labour', including a degree of 'specialisation', resurfaces again even in more generically defined roles. In practice the role envisaged here will likely be shaped more by some pre-existing professional agendas than by others (for example, by clinical rather than social agendas or vice versa).

This is not an abstract theoretical point. There are well-known contests about the construction of such roles. For example, the contests about how far the remits of 'health visitors', working with mothers of young babies, should be constructed around specific biomedically defined targets or by more open-ended and responsive agendas that arise out of the mothers' expressed concerns or social circumstances (Greenway and Entwistle, 2013). The crucial point here is that there is no universally agreed, or neutral, specification of what it is best to do for, or with, people – as discussed at length in earlier chapters; there can be tensions between different conceptions of what counts as good care and appropriate responsiveness to people. Health and social care professionals will not necessarily agree about what it is best to do for someone like Esther; indeed, on occasions it is quite possible that they will disagree about whether a specific line of 'care' is beneficial or harmful.

There has, for example, been an extensive amount of research into the factors that facilitate or inhibit 'inter-professional' working (Morrison and Glenny, 2012). This research is practically valuable because those setting out to build and sustain inter-professional partnerships can understand much more about the elements that need to be in place to optimise success – the importance of being explicit about and of negotiating around shared purposes; the development of joint protocols that set out the (flexible) division of tasks and responsibilities and mechanisms for conflict resolution; the advantages of some geographical co-location and inter-personal histories of trust and so on. Similarly, it is possible to flag up 'warning' factors that are likely to produce failures – the use of the language of partnership for 'public relations' reasons without proper investment of planning and resource, absence of joint working structures, and real or perceived power hierarchies or high levels of status-consciousness attached to strongly held professional identities (Hellawell, 2016).

But the body of research on inter-professional working is also theoretically illuminating. In exploring the conditions for effective partnership working it illuminates the contrasting sets of purposes motivating calls for greater integration. Integration can be driven by economic concerns – the search for system efficiency – and in that respect might be seen as but one of the myriad ways in which systems and institutions at all levels are under budget pressures to make continuous 'efficiency gains'. But it can also (and at the same time) be driven by an interest in improving the care of individuals and developing the collective knowledge and practice base needed for good care. The balance between these drivers can obviously make a difference to the ways in which it is pursued. Harris (2005) make a distinction here between 'instrumentalist partnership models' and 'learning partnership models' – seeing the former as tied to a 'what works' ideology arising from the generic operation of neoliberalism, unconstrained by local democratic participation or critique, and the latter as entailing a degree of local ownership and authentic engagement, and oriented towards exploring and debating 'what works'. Whereas the former seem to trade on 'certainty', the latter are built around uncertainty, recognising that effective partnerships between practitioners with different professional ideologies and conceptions of knowledge can only be attained through 'debate, argument, negotiation and bargaining' (Milbourne et al, 2003; Parrott, 2008).

These points about the different possible emphases shaping the agendas of professionals, as briefly illustrated by reference to health visitors, could be repeated for countless other examples. For instance it is manifest in relation to 'support for self-management' for people with long-term conditions, which is a paradigm example of an area where the integration of health and social care has conspicuous relevance and potential. A review of the literature in this area shows that multiple lenses can be applied and, in particular, that there are notable tensions between narrower biomedical and broader well-being conceptions of purpose (Morgan et al, 2017). Narrower approaches are oriented towards supporting people to 'manage their condition(s) well' and broader approaches to supporting them to 'manage well with their condition(s)'. Striking the right kinds of balances between helping someone to 'manage' a condition and helping them to lead the life they would like to lead is not easy. An individual health professional – working in dialogue with the person concerned – has to negotiate this tension between a narrower and broader emphasis and this can give rise to some difficult judgement calls and dilemmas (Entwistle et al, 2016). Social care professionals face similar dilemmas in their partnership working; and it is likely that – overall – there is a different pattern of emphases for health practitioners than for social care practitioners (given the salience of disease management for the former group).

These contrasting emphases of 'health work' and 'social work' are only one surface feature of deeper and broader differences in vantage points and practical orientations. For example, those who are used to working in community settings – whether in the traditions of social action, social work or social care – will tend to draw upon more inclusive conceptions of knowledge and purpose than do those who work in conventional healthcare. In so far as the latter aims to link up with and embrace the former – so that healthcare is better socially embedded and more widely shared – then it needs to relax its boundaries and extend its horizons. This broader compass includes a less prominent and more qualified place for individualist and biomedical norms: with more emphasis on building connections and communities; more explicit and official recognition of relative disadvantage (including patterns of discrimination and exclusion) as relevant to both understanding and action planning; an expectation that bringing individuals and groups together – as an end in itself and to make plans together – can itself form part of normal practice; a focus on ill-health as but one non-detachable aspect of people's identities and well-being needs and priorities; and a readiness to connect practice with other social and political agendas locally and nationally.

Of course there will also be considerable variations in outlook and norms among professionals in the same 'tribe' and significant overlaps in orientations between 'tribes'. However, the key thing to stress is that 'integrating' services or professions does not, in itself, in any fundamental way, resolve tensions or dilemmas about the 'right' (and ever shifting) balance between clinical and life priorities. In fact it can 'add in' a variety of other tensions as just outlined. But what it does do – which is something valuable but different – is open up new kinds of conversations and exchanges and broaden out the reference group within which these tensions might be both discussed and managed.

This is an absolutely critical point – which I will expand on below, and come back to in the next chapter. That is, bringing different parties together can eliminate some problems (most specifically those created by gaps or collisions in provision), and it can potentially provide a richer set of resources, including a better networked set of 'communities of practice' (Bridges et al, 2011; Ranmuthugala et al, 2011), to confront other more foundational problems (such as about the nature of good care or support) – providing that the conditions for teamwork and communication are in place. But, in many respects, it leaves these foundational problems about the nature of good care intact because they are not amenable to a logistical fix. Dialogue and collective deliberation are invaluable in these circumstances; but this is not because there is some technically correct answer waiting to emerge when all the data sources are lined up and harmonised but, rather, because they offer a way of collectively navigating and practically arbitrating between a range of credible, but inherently competing, perspectives and options. This is why I noted in Chapter One that Freida's puzzlement when faced with the priority-setting case can be understood as an essential step towards enlightenment. It is often better – more promising, more responsible – to be asking the right questions and to be stuck than to know how to proceed when asking the wrong questions.

The idea of integration needs to be unpacked. It points towards a number of different processes (and, implicit within those, a range of possible purposes). (i) From a 'systems' point of view integration means closer and more effective coordination between services. (ii) From the point of view of the individual being supported, integration means a less fragmented experience of care and the opportunity to actively pursue a more coherent life – and thereby, ideally, a means to underpin their own personal integration. (iii) From the point of view of practitioners it means both building new kinds of relationships with colleagues – as well as patients or service users – and being prepared to extend, revise, or at least critically reflect upon, one's own sense of role and role priorities. (iv) For all parties – lay and professional alike – it can represent the coming together of people to solve problems, to support one another, but also just to be and act together. Each of these four sets of concerns may sometimes be in tension with one another; and, as is too often the case in health policy-reform discourses, there is a danger that the challenges for people's personal and social identities and relations will be obscured by the emphases on system efficiency. Integration of care, in short, is a personal and social process as well as a system process. And we know from many other cases and settings that 'social integration' can be very testing and uncomfortable, and needs to be understood against the background of 'culture clashes', hierarchies of power and practices of exclusion. This means there must be big uncertainties about how, and how far, integration of care can close some of the deep-seated social divides between people, and their different social positions, forms of knowledge and purposes.

If integration is to work socially and epistemologically, then we have to develop and apply conceptions of integration that correspond with what Habermas calls 'communicative action' as well as 'strategic action', and that are guided by purposes of learning and the mutual understanding of diverse agents, and not only by institutional efficiency. Indeed an unqualified emphasis on strategic action for institutional efficiency is very likely to side-line the necessary dialogue and debate.

In summary, we need to be mindful of the distinctions between 'service integration' and 'social integration', and of what might be called 'assimilation' and 'coalition' versions of integration. The notion of assimilation indicates a striving for coherence and a uniformity of vision and practice. By contrast, the notion of coalition highlights the fact that joint working is about accommodation and compromise, and that it will encompass conflict as well as agreement. The former disguises tension, but the latter ensures it is visible. When it comes to working at the interface of different systems, institutions, professions and communities, including in the construction of new services and roles, assimilation models will tend to reproduce and extend the logic of some pre-existing service. However, coalition models will start from an acknowledgement that joint working is likely to be a messy business in which contrasting, and sometimes competing, logics have to find practical accommodations.

Clinical agendas can, and should be, used to support social agendas and vice versa. But it is equally the case that clinical and social agendas can sometimes pull in different directions and we cannot and should not make any general assumptions about which should have priority from case to case. Indeed much more than that is necessary – it is not enough to be agnostic about, or to aim to somehow be 'neutral' about, these competing purposes – we must strive to recognise and be ready to imaginatively respond to the qualitatively different ends, approaches and values that are embodied in clinical and social agendas.

Conclusion

In this chapter I have wanted to acknowledge and welcome something that has become a policy norm – that there are both system-wide efficiencies and 'person-centred' advantages in reformed cross-sectoral thinking and practice, including in the greater integration of health and social care systems. But I have also sought to point towards some of the practical limits to integration and the philosophical tensions between different conceptions of, elements of, and purposes served by, integration.

Before concluding I want to stress that these practical and philosophical constraints have very deep roots. Of course they reflect the problem of 'path dependency' – the fact that existing structures and cultures embody diverse historical currents that tend to reproduce themselves. They also reflect the fact that systems necessarily embody divisions of labour; divisions which are bound up with power hierarchies and with territorial and ideological disputes. There is, in short, scope for rich sociological explorations of how all of these factors create divergence and fragmentation and can inhibit integration. However, I would suggest, a full account of the limits to integration would combine an investigation of these sociological factors with an exploration of some of the philosophical factors that underpin them. Divisions between structures, cultures and practitioner groups may not be wholly defensible or logical. But neither are they wholly arbitrary or dispensable.

At base, the fragmentation of care arises because caring for people is itself inherently complex and contested – it requires us to engage both with multiple aspects of persons and with multiple kinds of goods, and also with disagreements about these things. The ultimate challenge for integration – I am suggesting – is not the one of 'holding together' divergent kinds of services or even divergent 'practice logics', but the one of 'holding together' divergent conceptions of what matters, and for whom. This is what I have sought to explore and illustrate in the last few chapters.

As discussed in Chapter Two – where I introduced the idea of 'responsiveness to persons' as a counterbalance to the biomedical model – this broad ideal orients us in a number of partly complementary, partly contrasting, ways. It is tempting to try to simplify the challenge by coming up with some relatively tidy version of 'person-centredness', for example, one focused on patient autonomy. But this will not carry us very far forward because it is itself restrictive and faces disputes about both its interpretation and its adequacy. If we are interested in people's well-being we also need to take seriously the implications of other characteristics of 'persons' discussed above – their subjectivity and 'inner life', including their capacity for suffering; their identities, histories and social contexts, including the way these are embedded in both personal and social relationships and social structures. This includes concerns about relative disadvantage, and various forms of structural inequality that underpin it, which can require us to look beyond individualist interpretations of personhood. Whether we are interested in ensuring that people have good health, or in promoting their well-being in some more general way, all of these dimensions are relevant.

The reasons why integration is challenging are thus not just practical ones (problems of logistics or social coordination). Rather, they reflect different stances (implicit theories) about what is good for people; how far carers should extend their gaze and involvement; which of various conceptions and dimensions of well-being should take precedence from case to case; when considerations of relative disadvantage or exclusion should frame our approaches, and so on. These disagreements are deep rooted because they arise not only from different readings of what may be good for people in particular cases but from different readings of what can and ought to count as good for people, and these rest upon philosophical commitments. That is, they represent different answers to ontological, epistemological and ethical puzzles about the nature of persons and personal well-being, and the bases on which, and confidence with which, we can make judgements about these things.

These philosophical tensions come to the surface and become visible, for example, in the conflicts that are familiar from attempts to increase inter-professional working (discussed above). Different professions are organised around specific sub-sets of problems and relevant goods, and operate with corresponding forms of knowledge, practical expertise and models of working and relating. However, once we understand integrated care more fully – in particular identifying the variety of forms of integration involved in bringing healthcare and social life closer together – it is evident not only that very many potential actors are implicated in integration but also that the locus of agency needed to achieve greater integration shifts significantly away from conventional professional roles. The fundamental challenge facing the integration of health and social care is that different paradigms cannot be 'integrated' without loss.

Nonetheless, the ambition to achieve greater integration is hugely important. It reflects and builds upon the crucial insight that health policy needs to attend to the underlying architecture of health and social care – to how both visions and practices of healthcare could better fit together. There is plenty of scope for accommodation, and a degree of merger, between paradigms, and there are countless opportunities for 'coalitions' between diverse agents. Strong systems of care (whether health systems or linked health and social care systems) will necessarily remain partly 'un-integrated' but will – by taking the aspiration and spirit of integration seriously – embrace contests between paradigms as productive and as opportunities for mutual learning.

Notes

[1] www.kingsfund.org.uk/audio-video/joined-care-sams-story.

[2] As told by Mats Bojestig on the Institute for Health Improvement's website – www.ihi.org/resources/pages/0069mprovementstories/ improvingpatientflowtheestherprojectinsweden.aspx.

[3] I am, for example, very grateful to have had the chance to visit the well-being services hosted by the Support and Information Centre at the UCL Cancer Centre (https://www.uclh.nhs.uk/OurServices/ServiceA-Z/Cancer/CSS/MCIC/Pages/ Home.aspx) and to be able talk through the idea of 'integrated care' with Hilary Plant.

SEVEN

Shaping the future

In this book I have been looking at some of the ways in which the currents of healthcare thinking have started to flow down different channels. New organising ideas have emerged that embody and produce different healthcare architectures and practice logics. I have relied on some very broad-brush terms to indicate these changes – the shift in emphasis from clinical to social lenses and agendas, including the relative decline in the dominance of the biomedical model and the growth of more person-centred models. Most of what I have said has raised concerns about these new emphases, and shown how they produce new problems or complications, but that is not meant to suggest that the trends I have been discussing should be resisted. (Certainly not – for the most part I want to cheer them along.) Rather, it is to stress that there are no problem-free paths in health policy, and to highlight, in particular, that there are normative tensions or 'value contests' built into any paths we might take.

In this chapter I will summarise some of the arguments of the book and draw some broad conclusions about the ongoing philosophical transition in health policy. There are signs of progress – for example, less presumed hierarchy between clinicians and the populations they serve and the growing acceptance that everyone can be seen as a health actor in a range of ways. In what follows I will explore some promising avenues for realising this more democratic conception of health-related action, especially around new ways of thinking about the spaces and resources that can support care. But there are also serious outstanding problems, most notably persisting health inequalities – and not only serious inequalities in health experiences but also inequalities in meaningful opportunities to be an effective healthcare actor.

This concluding chapter is necessarily broad ranging. I will begin by critiquing a 'delivery' paradigm of healthcare thinking and reiterating my contention that the philosophical transition is a transition 'towards philosophy'. In the main body of the chapter I will consider the importance of both 'digital health' and 'asset-based working' as potential paths forward, and I will then move on to reflect on the viability of making health a collective responsibility. Overall I want to argue that we are now required to think about health policy and healthcare in fundamentally different ways. This, I suggest, requires us to adopt a much more expansive and radical conception of a 'learning healthcare system'.

I am keen to displace, and in many places to dissolve or destroy, the tendency to think about healthcare as a question of 'delivery'. There can be a place for this notion but it is one that has a tendency to overrun the landscape like a deadly weed. At the professional–patient level we have become accustomed to the idea that the patient is not simply a destination to which healthcare is delivered. This insight has become familiar from work in healthcare ethics, on the evolving nature of healthcare professionalism, on quality and 'patient experience', and from work that highlights the nature of 'service goods' as contrasted with 'product goods'. But essentially the same insight – I am suggesting and will underline in this chapter – applies equally to health policies, systems and institutions across the board. The image or metaphor of 'delivery' fundamentally misses the point. At every level debates and questions about bringing about or achieving the 'goods' in question cannot be disentangled from debates and questions about what we think should be done and by whom, about what matters and about the nature of the relevant goods. Hence the focus of this book on the 'internal goods' of healthcare – crudely, 'health' and 'care' – and on the contests that arise when these goods are translated into either biomedical or/and person-centred categories and logics.

At the professional–patient level it is possible to do great harm if we 'deliver' something to an individual that does not accord with his or her values and preferences. Analogously it is potentially very harmful (and at scale) if we pursue health-policy ends driven by a commitment to 'what works', unless this is accompanied by an equal commitment to confronting very challenging debates and questions about what should count as working for the relevant stakeholders from case to case. The key thing to note is that neither 'health' nor 'care' is a clear-cut good; nor are they, in very many cases, goods that can be independently identified and packaged up by some for the benefit of others. Both the identification and realisation of these kinds of goods depend upon collaborative working, and on sometimes uncomfortable or difficult relationships between people with regard to both knowledge and action.

In concentrating my attention on policy transitions that relate to the internal goods of healthcare – about what, in general terms, healthcare is and is for – I have more or less neglected many other questions that are quite properly treated as relevant to the changing landscape of health policy. For example, I have not focused in on controversies about specific innovations – such as applications of stem cell therapy or gene editing and so on – or overlapping debates about what packages of specific treatments should be legally available, or how common resources should be allocated. Similarly I have neglected other questions that are central to health policy analysis; for example, although I have acknowledged the importance of questions about the appropriate balance between market and state forms of system coordination, I have said comparatively little about them.

Before continuing I should stress again that, despite their neglect here, questions about technological change or the social organisation of healthcare are very relevant to my theme. The goods of healthcare are shaped by many contextual factors, including the technological nexus and the networks of relationships and norms in which they are embedded. This is merely the corollary of the point that healthcare does not simply consist of separable 'products' that remain consistent and intact wherever they sit (like trays of nuts or bolts moving along conveyor belts). Hence even largely ignoring (important) questions about how efficient or equitable different models of provision are, we cannot afford to ignore related questions about their constitutive effects on healthcare goods. In relation to the 'market versus state' question, for example, these effects, although real, can sometimes be quite difficult to read, and subtle. There are crude generalisations and stereotypes in circulation – that markets are highly responsive to finely grained differences in preferences between people, or that they are merely a mechanism for getting vulnerable people to pay for things that they don't need or would be better off without; that state-organised collective provision is a way of underpinning the universal availability and quality of all worthwhile treatments, or that it is no more than an insensitive means of rationing 'bog standard' care. Except by underlining (as discussed, for example, in Chapter Four) the persuasive concerns that many have raised about the limits to market practices in healthcare, I am not interested in arbitrating between these kinds of generalisations. In practice we would need to look much more closely – both theoretically and empirically, and using methods that are sensitive to different contexts and cases – at how the milieux in which healthcare is enacted shape the ways in which various healthcare goods are interpreted and realised and in which healthcare is lived and experienced. In addition, as I will go on to argue later in the chapter, we need to look beyond the state 'versus' market debate, or even questions about the contribution of a 'third sector', and ask how the coordination of healthcare can reflect the more democratic aspirations embedded in reforming currents. Indeed the issue of the mix of state, market and 'third sector' organisation is only one very general example of the social construction of healthcare goods. Overlapping analyses can and should be applied to the constitutive effects of different kinds of institutional regimes, approaches to management, models of professionalism and so on – in every case social milieux shape healthcare goods.

Healthcare goods as social goods

The philosophical transition I have looked at – which can be summarised very roughly as the rise of a social conception of healthcare – can be described in contrasting ways and deployed in different stories. One story is a straightforwardly positive account of policy progress in which the healthcare agenda has been enlarged to enable more respect for, and responsiveness to, persons, including more attention to the broader social determinants of health. But there is a contrasting story – less straightforward, and more problematic to evaluate – according to which the philosophical transition 'muddies the waters' of healthcare, that is, produces fuzzier categories and ever-increasing contestability and uncertainty. These two stories are not wholly incompatible with one another; indeed I am inclined to subscribe to both of them. But they do not sit together entirely comfortably because they highlight different things. The former is useful for indicating general policy directions and aspirations; but the latter underlines the many complexities and balancing acts generated by attempts to translate these general aspirations into real-world policy and practice decisions. In this section I will develop this point and say more about how these two stories – positive and problematising – are connected.

I have adopted the language of 'person-centred care' to illustrate and discuss the philosophical transition in earlier chapters. But the same themes can be briefly summarised, albeit at quite an abstract level, by sticking with the underlying idea that there is a shift in emphasis from clinical to social concerns (that is, where 'concerns' includes both social matters and social perspectives).

If we place a lot of weight on clinical agendas, and interpret these in terms of the management of disease, or the pursuit of other biomedically defined outcomes, then there is at least a plausible case for being able to make relatively value-free, impersonal or 'objective' claims about what we are doing. (Noting, of course, that there are important contests even here relating to the socio-cultural constitution, organisation and exercise of clinical knowledge.) This is because the claims we are making refer largely to bodies or to other biophysical or biochemical entities. However, the moment we move away from this focus things become more uncertain and contested, and each step further away that we move, the more this process accelerates until it soon becomes quite dizzying.

For any single individual, having their biological constitution moved closer to a state that might 'objectively' correspond with what is 'normal' or 'clinically healthy' for them may or may not be desirable – depending upon the broader costs and benefits entailed and on their other projects and commitments. The values of individuals determine what counts as 'good' or 'bad' here; and this is now an uncontroversial thing to say, even if it is not always easy to operationalise in practice (which involves ensuring proper mutual communication, understanding and reliable identification of values and so on). One (rough) way to handle this 'incursion' of individual values and preferences in the case of relatively immediate treatment decisions is to envisage a practical split between clinical 'facts' and personal 'values', and to see the latter as an important extra consideration, and 'veto', to the former. But this tactic becomes much harder, and eventually unsustainable, as we broaden the frame of reference along one or both of two axes. Specifically, that is, if (i) we look at broader time–space continua (for example at policies that affect more than one person, especially system or population-level judgements); or (ii) we consider broader conceptions of health and health-related action, including both the range of conditions underpinning, and various manifestations of, health.

Firstly, there is a high level of uncertainty and contestability attached to broad-based policy claims; for example, claims about health system organisation, health service design or health promotion. And this is not simply because of difficulties of making causal judgements, in relatively open-ended social systems, about what would happen if x or y is done, but also because the lenses through which we make such judgements, or the categories that we use in constructing them, are heavily value laden. In addition we are, at the same time, seeking to be responsive to numerous people who will often have very different sets of values and preferences. Secondly, once we acknowledge that claims about health may not solely be claims about biological states of affairs but might be about other aspects of health-related quality of life – such as how people experience illness, how far they are (enabled to) engage in matters that affect them (clinically or more broadly), the quality of relationships and trust they experience with carers, the overall satisfaction they have with their lot, and whether the opportunities are in place for them to be able to have a life they regard as fulfilling, and so on – then it becomes obvious that there are multiple and competing value-laden conceptions of what might and should count in organising or assessing healthcare. In short, a shift in emphasis from clinical to social concerns moves us towards a heavily contested arena in which potential controversies abound and value tensions become the norm.

Thus, as I briefly indicated in the opening chapter, we are arguably talking about a philosophical transition in two senses. The opening up of agendas and complexities – as the centre of gravity of health policy has gradually shifted to embrace broader conceptions of healthcare, including health-related action and goods – amounts to a philosophical transition in the sense of a shift in underlying 'philosophies' of healthcare. But, I want to say, this can also be seen as a transition towards 'philosophy'. That is, the emerging world of health policy is one that demands the management of pervasive disagreements about what matters (including the categories we should be operating with, and the voices that should determine this) and the continuous negotiation of normative tensions. These broadly philosophical issues are not a 'side show', or an extra layer of considerations occurring alongside strategic, regulatory and technical questions about service organisation or 'good practice'; rather, they are inseparable from these questions and sit at the heart of them.

My argument, in summary, has been that while each strand of person-centred thinking provides a fundamentally important counterweight to narrow framings of healthcare, and can be defended in these terms, they each also take us into difficult territory. Bluntly speaking, they cannot simply be treated as providing 'solutions' to the shortcomings of biomedically dominated healthcare. This is for a variety of reasons, which I will pull together into three points.

First, in each case there is some value to be attached to the more traditional and narrower emphases, and some grounds to defend them. This leaves a question of how to combine and balance the narrow and broader emphases. Second, in each case there are many possible interpretations of what is meant by, and entailed by, the reference to 'persons' and the aspect of person-centredness that is foregrounded. That is, there are multiple contests of interpretation to be had both within and across the strands discussed in Chapters Three, Four and Five. A key axis here is how far 'persons' should be read in an individualist way, that is, as relating to persons as separate, or in more social ways, that is, as relating to persons as related and socially embedded. Third, overlapping with the first two points, there are no clear means of agreeing how much of what kinds of these 'counterweights' are for the good. In other words, it is not simply that the kinds of 'corrections' that are pointed to are open to considerable interpretation but also that they can be the subject of legitimate and conscientious disagreements going well beyond the arena of technical judgement. In these three points, and in the preceding chapters, I have sketched out a large matrix of contestation.

A simple way of summarising some of the contests here is to ask whether there is any case that could be mounted for (rather than just against) the social authority of professionals, the management of diseases or the standardisation of provision in healthcare. Clearly the answer, in relation to each of the three strands, is yes. Advocates of these things could easily produce principled arguments to support their positions. Furthermore, no one (or at least, virtually no one) is suggesting that these things don't have a place or that the arguments that could be rehearsed for them could be wholly rejected. For example, the roles of doctors (and health professional roles more broadly) may need to adapt, they may even need to be substantially reconfigured, but advocates of person-centred approaches are not suggesting that they should disappear altogether. And part of the core rationale of professional roles is that professionals are licensed to exercise specific kinds of expertise-based social authority. Given this, there are limits to how far it is meaningful, sensible or morally defensible for health professionals to subjugate their judgement to other people's preferences or demands. This seems relatively non-contentious. However, this leaves scope for very widespread disagreements about quite how, and how extensively, we should reconceptualise the professional–patient relationship, and how best – in various respects – to combine professional and patient (or lay, public and so on) agency and authority.

It is arguably this reconceptualisation of relationship – and indeed the intensified emphasis on relationship – that is the central issue here. Health services and professionals, in, for example, deciding on the relative emphasis to be given to disease management and/or standardised protocols and practices, need to work in dialogue with the people they serve and to be responsive (among other things) to what matters to people. Indeed – as I will go on to explore further in the following sections – most fundamentally they need to find ways of collaborating with and working alongside individuals and communities, that is, ways of working *with* people and not just *for* or *on* them. Both for these reasons and as an end in itself services and professionals need to build relationships. This marks a change from a transactional or 'delivery' paradigm and this inevitably also moves us onto a landscape where instrumentalist and technicist categories, centred on outcomes, effectiveness and efficiency, are inadequate. In the emerging landscape some degree of comfort in dealing with personal and social values, and associated value contests, has become an 'essential requirement' in the job descriptions of all policy makers and professionals.

The fact that emerging ideas – and the value contests that attach to them – make both policy making and analysis complicated does not mean that we cannot come to any substantive conclusions about policy directions. It is rather that we have to be mindful of the complications and contests that arise when we seek to interpret and apply these conclusions in practice. For example, I would argue, based on the ground I have covered, that any defensible interpretation of person-centredness needs to be 'plural'. That is, that it should both reflect the multi-faceted nature of persons (not reducing person-centred thinking to one dimension) and – equally vital – be alive to the reality of people in communities, and as collectives, and not just to individual persons considered separately. If people are to be able to enjoy health, and participate in health-related practices and policies, there needs to be a heavy emphasis on structural action towards building better health ecologies for the common good. And this should not be seen as simply about 'public health' in a restricted sense but as applying equally to the systems that underpin social well-being, including healthcare services. Good healthcare depends upon 'integrated' attention to the social and material conditions of our lives, including the organisation of effective healthcare systems and services. This is not in any way to reject the importance of personalised attention to, and biographical working with, individuals. It is vital – although not necessarily easy – to ensure that these things are not squeezed out by system designs and priorities. But, while recognising this, it should be clear that these individually oriented forms of person-centred care actually depend upon us acting holistically and collectively, and crafting systems accordingly.

These, by way of 'headlines', are some of my own substantive conclusions. However, to repeat, I fully appreciate that the translation of these broad ideas into practical reality will be both challenging and contested. In the reminder of this chapter I consider some of these complications.

Person power – digitally delivered?

One of the most clear-cut trends in policy thinking is the ever-growing recognition of the importance of patients and populations as health-related actors. This basic idea lies behind diverse developments such as self-management, co-design of health services, patient-led research or education, community development partnerships, health-related social media fora and so on. The notion that everyone is a health actor is one example of the process, which I have referred to from time to time, of challenging or 'inverting' limited traditional norms. In this case, for example, it can be accompanied by sentiments and statements (or slogans) to the effect that healthcare is becoming more equal or more democratic. This broadly 'democratising' current is an absolutely key dimension of the philosophical transition I am reviewing. It is not just that the focus of healthcare is expanding to include the whole social realm but that the locus of agency is increasingly seen as spread across the social realm. It is also important, however, to note that a range of different things are encompassed by referring to people as health actors. At minimum this includes the notion of people acting for themselves in relation to disease management – as clinical co-decision makers, self-carers and so on. It also, importantly, includes the myriad ways in which people initiate, contribute to and organise forms of mutual or collective care giving, not least by participating in 'third sector' activities. But, most generally, it should clearly signal the contribution of the same individuals as co-citizens and thereby 'policy actors' having a say over the shape of, and participating in, all aspects of the broader health and social care ecology. While acknowledging this range we should, of course, bear in mind that there can sometimes be problems in combining these different kinds of agency – people cannot always wear 'multiple hats' at the same time. Similarly, it is important to be aware of these different kinds of agency if we are collectively interested in providing the conditions for, or supporting, people's agency – there is, in short, a difference between fostering the 'activation' of patients to look after themselves and fostering the 'activism' of community members to reshape their health and healthcare landscapes. (I will return to this idea shortly.)

However, welcoming an expanded conception of health action is not enough. As I set out in Chapter One, important reforming ideas – including the idea that we are all health-related actors – need to be embodied in new social and/or technological practices if they are to be advanced beyond rhetoric or aspiration. It is typically the 'socio-material translation' of ideas that marks the real shifts that are being called for rather than the mere articulation of them. Similarly, it is the failure to achieve socio-material translation that means that even the very best reforming aspirations are often only ever partly or patchily implemented. As we saw in the last few chapters it is relatively easy to create a 'rhetorical shift' – we can, for example, disseminate the idea that patients should share decisions, or that professionals need to act 'holistically' or in coordinated ways, or that communities should co-produce their own care. But once we engage more fully with such ideas we become conscious that exactly what is entailed by them is unclear and disputed, and that we may lack the relationships and structures or any obvious route map for translating them into practice. Aspirations to shift the 'organising ideas' of healthcare actually require both ontological and epistemological shifts – changes in the nature of the relationships and structures that underpin healthcare and in the kinds of expertise that are treated as valuable and are drawn upon in determining and evaluating good practice.

If we want to move beyond rhetoric the 'depth' of change needed is substantial. This can be illustrated using a very crude analogy. We can imagine that a group of people who occupy a building and who are served by a vending machine find the machine unsatisfactory – for example, because it has a restricted range of options that seem to be determined by someone else and not by them. They meet and brainstorm and consider what else the vending machine could dispense. Using great ingenuity they gradually expand the range of options. This eventually includes allowing people to purchase tokens that can be exchanged for a much wider range of snacks and meals that they can obtain or prepare themselves and install in their own communal fridges. In this case it is obvious that there are severe limits to how much can be achieved by sticking with the vending-machine model. What eventually comes about and is successful is a model where the vending machine fades into the background and is overshadowed by something much more like communal food preparation and sharing (akin to that practised in a Sikh temple or Gurdwara). It is far too simplistic to say that dominant healthcare practices are comparable to a vending machine; but it is fair to say that many current policy aspirations require a similar depth of structural change.

If substantial – not just limited and patchy – healthcare change is to be accomplished, in a way that does some degree of justice to changes in health-policy rhetoric, then we need both new ways of thinking and new ways of acting – that is, *both* new organising ideas or logics *and* new practices that embody these ideas. Plausible candidates for both these things are 'asset-based' working and 'digital health'. These both represent potentially foundational shifts in our understanding of basic categories, including, not least, the assumptions we make about what counts as 'resources' and 'space'.

'Asset-based' working (Rippon and Hopkins, 2015) provides another clear example of 'inverted thinking' – instead of simply constructing the public as a whole, or specific communities and individuals as representing a 'burden of care' for the health system, it suggests that we should think of them as system assets. People can and do look after themselves and one another, and they might be better encouraged and supported to do so, with considerable mutual benefits to both services and populations. The growth of peer-led self-management support groups is a clear example of the potential in this area. A label such as 'asset-based' is simply a more generalised and systematic way of capturing the very many multiple ways of thinking about people as actors (alluded to in previous chapters and listed above) and, of course, as actors who are intimately bound up with day-to-day health experiences and practices – it both crystallises and promotes the necessary 'gestalt switches' in policy thinking.

Digital health is an even more high-profile example of potential foundational change. Asset-based approaches and digital health are both future-oriented themes (and not wholly rhetorical tropes but themes that have fostered examples of practice change). There are many overlaps between them but, on the surface, they seem to stress very different things – for example, the former might be seen as de-medicalising, or as involving the transcendence of biomedical thinking through, for example, community development work, whereas the latter, at least superficially, highlights technology-led change and the further spread of biomedicine. I will discuss the promise of digital health further in the remainder of this section and return to some of the implications and complications of asset-based approaches in the following sections.

One version of an imagined future of diffused health action and self-care – including yet another classic example of inversion – arises from the pervasiveness of 'high tech' resources in the everyday lives of people because of the near-ubiquity in affluent societies of the smartphone and associated applications. It can be found, for example, in the best-selling book by Eric Topol, *The Patient Will See You Now* (2015), which charts and celebrates the rise of digital health as the vehicle that finally liberates the patient from professional domination. Topol's is a very bracing account – thought provoking and thoughtful as well as popular and upbeat – of the reconfigurative effects on healthcare of technological and social change. It discusses seemingly science-fiction futures morphing into the mundane present. The quantity of biomedical data – from molecular to environmental levels – that can be digitally captured, tracked and speedily processed for, and potentially by, each individual means that medicine can now be directed towards and by 'digitised persons'. For healthcare institutions and clinicians this potentially brings about dramatic advantages in the collection and utilisation of data, not only offering efficiencies in an aggregative sense but also offering the ability to be digitally responsive to individuals in their myriad differences. However, these developments also have potentially dramatic implications for the agency of patients, carers and other service users. For example, they potentially mean not only people being able to have ready access to lab tests, scans and records but also, in many cases, being able to generate tests, make diagnoses and monitor key biomedical markers themselves with the support of readily available devices. Digital technology means that they are also increasingly able to seek professional clinical advice online, and in a variety of ways that suit them. Overall, these shifts, it is suggested, will completely change the centre of gravity of healthcare.

Topol's treatment of the pace and significance of potential changes in practices and expectations, although some will it see as exaggerated, deserves to be taken seriously. It offers a stimulating 'thought experiment' about the ways in which norms can both be preserved by, and radically disrupted by, socio-material factors, including technological developments. There is no doubt that smartphones, along with the internet and digital communications more generally, are changing the way people live their lives and reworking expectations in many areas both inside and outside of healthcare. In any treatment of the future of health policy this is an area that requires attention; but it is also, for me, another way of approaching and reviewing some of the foundational changes that I have been considering in this book. In particular it can be used to highlight questions about how far-reaching and radical the shift in the locus of agency, away from policy makers and professionals and towards people and communities, might be and should be.

Topol's account is significant because it shows quite clearly why the power of biomedicine and the power of doctors should not be equated, or why the transfer of influence, authority and control to non-medical actors is not the same as de-medicalisation (as signalled in Chapter Three). Rather, one way of conceiving of the diffusion of, or transfer of, power away from health professionals is precisely to see it as a transfer of biomedical knowledge and action to patients and populations. Shifting the locus of control of biomedicine to patients might be seen as a paradigm example of *both* 'person centred' thinking *and* medicalisation. Topol describes this as representing a potentially decisive shift away from the concentration of authority and power in the hands of privileged experts – what he calls 'eminence-based medicine' – and towards 'democratic' healthcare.

In some senses this is plausible. If the information revolution, including the miniaturisation of diagnostic monitoring technologies and so on, brings about much more ready, and much more equal, access to clinical data and clinical knowledge, then the idea of the 'expert patient' is extended or transformed. It may increasingly come to mean not just someone who has an 'inside knowledge' of their own health experiences and medical histories but someone who also has access to both relatively specialist equipment and a solid clinical understanding of their conditions. But although this can be seen as 'democratising' in one important sense there are other senses of 'democratic' according to which this claim would be much more contentious.

The (not extravagantly named) 'digital revolution' almost seems designed to produce 'escape velocity' for the social diffusion of healthcare beyond clinical arenas as traditionally and narrowly conceived. It allows for many of the concerns of the clinic to be enacted, attended to and made salient anywhere and everywhere. Digital developments facilitate new forms of relationship, collaboration and learning for professionals, patients and populations separately or in combination. They can be seen as enabling 'person-centred' advances in key respects; specifically they provide substantially enhanced scope for the agency of non-professional actors and for flexibility of action and response. In other words, these technological advances mean that individuals and communities should be able to participate more fully in a healthcare system that is also more personalised. Obviously these potential advantages are being indicated here 'in principle' and the extent to which they are meaningfully realised depends upon looking at specific examples in varying contexts. But there are good reasons for optimism in many respects.

Of course – as always – there are also worries about the rise of digital health. It is important to acknowledge these, even if only to try to steer developments so as to minimise their chances of materialising. I will briefly rehearse three of them here – all of which can be seen to problematise, and cast into doubt, the notion that the centrifugal forces of digitisation are democratising.

First, there are plausible concerns about whether some of these developments should properly be viewed as an intensification of 'medicalisation' in a pejorative sense. Here the worry is that the close texture of everyday life could be 'colonised', through smartphone or similar devices, by biomedical categories and that, despite a degree of willing participation and even some enthusiasm, this may entail some significant (and ultimately unwelcome) distortion of people's life-worlds. In other words, rather than a take-over of biomedicine by 'ordinary folk', what we might be witnessing is more a take-over of people's ordinary lives by biomedicine, including corporate biomedical agencies. In this case one of the things we are being encouraged to be wary of is a powerfully seductive 'healthism' that is incompatible with broader notions of personal well-being. (This is, of course, parallel to other widely discussed fears – or perhaps 'moral panics' – about the digital world stimulating, for example, narcissism or addiction, or super-charged hypochondria.)

Concerns of this sort rest upon two premises, each of which might be investigated, questioned and qualified in the light of both empirical and ethical considerations. They rest on the premise that the organising principles of digital health just reproduce the reductionism and 'partial sightedness' of biomedicine; and on the premise that in so far as people seem to embrace such 'partial sightedness' they either are ambivalent about it or – when they are positive – may subsequently discover that they have made a mistake (that is, are wrong about what they think they value). I do not propose to assess the strength of these assumptions here, and to do so would not be straightforward. In principle, digitisation – given the immense storage and analytic potential of computing – makes it possible for both patients and professionals to record and share a much wider spectrum of information – for example, related to preferences and values as well as life-style, and life-context factors, including personalised 'narrative information' – in ways which would previously have been inconceivable. And the extent to which people do (or ought) to value having ongoing access to, and reminders of, biomedical (and other) data about themselves, when this might be more or less useful or threatening (or both), raises a particularly demanding set of questions, which I will leave on one side. However, any serious consideration of these matters would start from the notion that it 'depends on how it is done'. We would need to consider – across a variety of cases – what or who is driving, shaping and taking part in the changes before coming to any conclusions about how person-responsive, liberatory or democratising they are. This takes me on to other worries.

Second, there are worries about the 'digital divide' – the fear that digital health developments leave some people behind and exacerbate health inequalities. Digital health may help to flatten the hierarchies between professionals and patients but it can create other hierarchies. As is well understood, not everyone has equal resources or capabilities to take advantage of the information revolution. These disparities could be partly off-set by collective provision, but to the extent that emerging initiatives are supported by individuals having their own 'digital infrastructure' (for example, easy and multiple points of access to the web) and associated skills and confidence, this will not be an arena of equal access to care. In the first instance, in a period of early adopters, the resulting inequalities may not be particularly pernicious. However, there are reasons to worry that their significance could grow and become substantial. The risk is not merely that some sections of the population may acquire the means and dispositions to adopt digital health practices effectively while others do not, but also that as new forms of monitoring, communication, patient education and self-care are diffused other, more traditional, forms of care and support will be reduced or withdrawn, disproportionately affecting the most disadvantaged.

This leads to a third worry. The concern about inequalities is not limited to a concern about equal access to emerging technologies. The same disparities and hierarchies apply in relation to participation in the design, organisation and regulation of such technologies. The issue is not just who uses things, but who shapes things. Any credible claim that digital advances (or any other currents in health policy) are democratising ones must depend upon this. Of course we could say, for example, that giant supermarket chains are relatively 'democratic' – as contrasted with some exclusive jewellery shop in Knightsbridge, London – in the sense that they serve the mass of the people; but this does not mean that they are run on, or embody, democratic principles. Although there are grounds for scepticism here, determining the relevance and seriousness of this worry is, again, not clear cut.

The digital revolution does contain egalitarian, including communitarian, possibilities – it should not be seen purely through individualist, consumerist (or biomedical) lenses – but claims that it is democratising certainly cannot go unchallenged. Prainsack (2017) helpfully distinguishes between different models of 'empowerment' that have relevance here – and indeed across the board – individual, instrumental, democratic and emancipatory models. The first two models refer to the personal and system-level benefits of enabling and 'harnessing' individual choice. The latter two models conceive of empowerment in social terms – as broadening the space for broader processes of policy inclusion, deliberation and decision making, and – most radically – as people working to actively resist dominant categories, 'take back' power and define their own experiences and contexts (women's health movements being a paradigm case). This taxonomy is a more careful elaboration of the rough distinction I made earlier between 'activation' and 'activism'. We should be ready to interrogate, and make these kinds of critical discriminations about, all reform efforts that make claims about empowerment or liberation, both in and beyond digital health.

Having noted these reservations and limitations, the rise of digital health does seem to be a critical development in the philosophical transition I have been charting. It provides a whole new axis for the social-material translation of ideas such as self-management, co-production and so on; that is, those ideas that are central to the realisation of person-centred models of healthcare. Furthermore, digital developments can clearly work as 'disruptive technologies' – helping to challenge, dislodge and replace some of the sedimented practices and habits associated with traditional biomedical relationships. This is an important element of overcoming policy path dependency (because, unless we can see and find ways to build alternative paths, we will naturally stick with the well-worn ones.) Perhaps most significantly, given the simplifying lens I have been using in this book, the digital realm arguably represents a 'new space' both between and beyond the 'clinical world' and the 'social world'.

Cyberspace might be seen as part neither of the clinical realm nor of the social realm, or might be seen as both at the same time. New spaces (even in the prosaic sense of physical meeting places and so on) are often critical for reforging healthcare relationships. The indefinitely large and adaptable realm of cyberspace has indefinitely large potential to create new patterns of relationships and to rework power hierarchies. It can be a shared space where patients and clinicians can meet in new ways, and it can be a space where patients and publics share and build knowledge (including through their own rigorous research), organise themselves and challenge conventional structures and understandings. There are countless possibilities. But obviously we cannot make lazy assumptions about the magical (or even benign) power of digital 'solutions'. All of the things that are a source of concern about the wrong directions that biomedicine can take still have relevance in cyberspace. As noted above, we need, for example, to be ready to ask critical questions about the ownership, control or steering of hardware, software and digital activity.

In summary, the advances arriving, and promised, here can in many key respects be seen to ally with the rise in person-centred thinking. However, in welcoming this we need to attend to the multiple dimensions and contestability of person-centredness. In particular the discussion of equality and democracy above reintroduces questions about the relationship between the 'individual person' and the 'social person'. As discussed in Chapter Four, attention to the personal aspects of healthcare can direct us (inwards) to the individual biography and life-world, or (outwards) towards the inter-personal, cultural and social 'materials' out of which such biographies or life-worlds are forged. The latter positively invites questions about concerns such as health inequalities, solidarity, democracy and the 'liberatory potential' of socio-technological change; the former can easily obscure them or bracket them out. Indeed it is plausible that in the majority of cases the advocacy of person-centred trends – including those that foreground agency, holism and personalisation as I have – does not really disrupt some of the core categories of biomedicine as a professional–client activity but 'carries over' and relies on individualist assumptions. In these instances person-centredness still means conceiving of healthcare as broadly consisting of transactions between individual professionals and patients, but simply imagining that these transactions will change their character. These assumptions – of 'methodological individualism' – are one of the things I have tried to problematise and push against in the exploration of person-centredness offered in this book.

Reducing power hierarchies between professionals and patients, and enabling patients or patient advocates – as individuals – to be more active, can be presented as a very important shift in assumptions about healthcare. But questions about the many other broader forms of inequality cannot be side-lined. This is not just because they are ethically and politically important in their own right, but also for reasons summarised in the previous section. Most health policy decisions – whether expressly about healthcare or about factors that affect health – cannot be disaggregated into individual or 'private' decisions. They affect more than one person – and often very many people – are value-laden and require the application of social lenses. If we have a commitment to the idea that people should participate in matters that affect them, and that people's own values, preferences and involvement are relevant to good decision making and practice, then it follows that we need to pay some attention to inequalities of participation. If there are seriously unequal opportunities for participation within a health system, then it cannot be viewed as a good one.

Collective responsibility for health: asking too much?

The imagined future implicit in the transition I have been discussing is one in which health and healthcare are a collective responsibility. This is not to say that there is no room in such a world for professionals, or those charged with special responsibilities. (The next section is based on the assumption that such people have a vital role, and will explore the implications of that further.) It is simply what follows from various well-established trends. Relevant expertise is now seen as widely distributed – not only 'lay' expertise about what people value, or about how policies affect people, but also some formerly restricted kinds of biomedical expertise. In addition, the social turn in healthcare means that what counts as the knowledge base for health policy has expanded – for example, making the humanities and social sciences (along with other less formal and 'academic' approaches to human and social understanding) much less marginal. More generally, the normative climate is one in which hierarchies of influence and authority are being gradually eroded. Above all, the recognition that healthcare policy judgements are intrinsically and substantially judgements about values and negotiating values means both (a) that specialist technical expertise – although still vitally important – has a clearly circumscribed contribution to make in many instances, and (b) that broader forms of engagement and participation are a requirement both for valid decision making and for sufficiently broad-ranging action.

But collective responsibility seems to be asking a lot. I have been arguing that the health-policy agenda has proliferated in many different ways – that it needs to be sensitive to people's life-worlds and biographies; that the social context of health is a crucial consideration and that this entails an explosion of relevant factors to consider; that policy judgements require literacy about values and the continuous balancing of competing values across many different axes. However, at the same time and for the same reasons, I am suggesting that we are, and need to be, shifting across from a 'top-down' to a more diffused approach to policy making and health-related action. The more complex things get, I am suggesting, the less we should leave things to the experts (or, more precisely, to the forms of expertise that have traditionally been privileged). We would be foolish if this combination of suggestions did not give us pause – especially given the prevalence of structural and cultural disadvantage reiterated in the previous section.

Although on a larger scale, and complicated by scale and diversity, many of the issues here are closely analogous to the ones that arise at the individual level when we are encouraged to 'look after ourselves' and to 'share decisions'. Specifically, there are questions about how far people are able, and feel able, to take on new responsibilities; about tensions in relation to what counts as evidence or relevant knowledge; and about how collective decision making and action is practically accomplished. There are well-known extra complications when we move from decision making by individual patients to considering group decision making; for example, that the latter can generate many more 'contradictions', given competing demands from different people, and even – at least on simplistic constructions of direct democracy, which roughly equates to voting – competing demands at the collective level when whole groups can strongly support two incompatible things at the same time.

Just as at the level of the individual, there are some unavoidable normative tensions built into participatory or social action models of health policy making and policy enactment. For example, there is a need to think about how systems and services can both be responsive to people's agency and also support and practically mediate that agency. There are obvious dangers of a 'free for all', especially in the many real-world settings where the loudest voices, or the best-connected voices, are most influential. Not everyone who is bound up with healthcare is equally well placed to make a contribution to it. While accepting that all people have relevant expertise, we must also recognise that not all forms of relevant expertise are evenly distributed. Neither, of course, are all forms of environmental, physical and emotional security, or economic or social capital, or (as a result) personal or social capabilities, or, for that matter, physical and mental health (the absence of which makes people vulnerable and sometimes relatively powerless). There are profoundly difficult and delicate balances to be struck here. On the one hand, it is possible to talk about supporting people's agency but, as a result of poor practice, to in effect demean, dismiss or patronise them. On the other hand, it is possible to seek to engage and empower people but, as a result, to make unreasonable demands on them and thereby effectively abandon them to the margins. In so far as the diffusion of agency is seen as being about a wider distribution of responsibility, then we need to be alive to the possibility of its becoming either unduly burdensome or simply unjust. (This is analogous to the worries about 'off-loading' responsibility to individual patients in the narrow models of shared decision-making discussed in Chapter Three.)

What is called for is something analogous to the 'both/and' approach that emerged in the earlier discussion of Mol's 'logic of care'. This means, for example, rejecting simplistic constructions of people as either dependent or independent (for example, either passive recipients of care or sovereign individuals and so on) but, by contrast, accepting that we are all of us always both relatively dependent and relatively independent (with different balances at different times). Our autonomy is relational – it both deserves to be respected and needs to be supported. Understanding that expressions and exercises of autonomy are socially produced, and sometimes self-consciously co-produced, is not to note a shortcoming in autonomy but to understand its nature. In some contexts it makes sense to operate as if individuals are separate sovereign individuals (for example, when they are shopping or voting) but we do not always have to see things like that. This is especially relevant in healthcare, which is – to repeat, for one final time, about both care and health.

Health policy, whether seen as a top-down enterprise or as about 'looking after ourselves', is not only about 'decisions' directed towards health outcomes. It must encompass an interest in broader processes of communication and mutuality, in how we treat one another, in caring relationships and in avoiding the neglect of people who are disadvantaged with regard to their immediate or prospective health needs. The decisions–outcomes distinction thus needs to be problematised in this context. It is not entirely irrelevant to an arena of diffused health action but it is too crude and imports a technicist and reductionist mind-set (from the biomedical model). People can look after one another partly by simply being together and taking an interest in one another – if we had to cash them out in technicist terms, these forms of mutuality are simultaneously 'collecting data', 'making decisions' and 'intervening'. In other words, mutuality is both a means and an end – it constitutes care or solidarity but it also builds otherwise unattainable detailed knowledge that might underpin further action.

Mutual care and community responsibility are not just idealised abstractions but are being embodied in real-world practical initiatives. For example, there are a number of emerging initiatives that bring together ideas and practices based on asset-based community action – these initiatives consciously aim for the integration of public health, community development, health services and voluntary action. Some of these are relatively local developments aimed to bring communities together to promote health and provide, for example, dementia-friendly and non-obesogenic climates and environments.[1] But they can also be large-scale, regional, system-level reforms designed to utilise community assets to help integrate and improve services and well-being across the board. For example, Greater Manchester's ambitious Health and Social Care Partnership aims to bring together prevention, community care and hospital services around the principles of social action, inter-sectoral partnership, support for carers, health equity, co-production and person-centredness.[2] In this vision community-based assets are recognised and built such that diverse actors are enabled to embrace the challenge of, and share the burden of, mutual care. Key to these developments is the notion that healthcare, and decisions about healthcare, are not just 'done by some' but belong, and need fostering, at the level of everyone's everyday life.

There is, in addition, nothing to stop people assigning many areas of decision making to other people. This is the norm and has many advantages. Indeed it would be difficult to make sense of the idea that everyone should be directly involved in all the decisions that affect them. To ask for this would be to ask for the practically impossible –

both logistically and psychologically. For a start, we may choose to leave decisions largely to other people: when their effects on us are trivial (I may be quite fussy about the food I order, but pay little attention to the choice of plate it comes on); or when someone else has been down the same or a similar road before and has relevant experience (I may happily defer when it comes to the choice of wine, given my relative inexperience and my confidence in my friends' awareness of my preferences). Most expressions of collective (including democratic) decision making are indirect expressions – we collectively assign responsibilities to specific sets of people and we have various formal and informal mechanisms to support, monitor and, when we feel let down by them, challenge such people.

More emphasis on collective responsibility – which I take to be a crucial feature of emerging approaches to health policy – need not radically change the balance between direct and indirect decision making. But, I would argue, it does entail some changes to this balance, along with substantial changes in the way indirect decision making is understood and should work. Given the fact that an effective health system is not only meant to serve the interests of many but actually depends upon the involvement and recognition of indefinitely large numbers of health actors, then anyone who serves as a representative decision maker has a double obligation to be richly informed about and properly responsive to system stakeholders. And this kind of responsiveness need not be simply a vague ideal because there are normatively based and practical approaches that have been developed to help operationalise these ideals and to overcome the dangers of a 'free for all' or of the simplistic forms of direct democracy mentioned above. Most notable here is the work developed under the rubric of 'deliberative democracy' (Bohman and Rehg, 1997; Thompson, 2008). There are a family of approaches here with different theoretical undercurrents and different practical methods (such as Citizens' Juries, Consensus Conferences and Deliberative Focus Groups), but what they broadly share in common is a concern for a collection of data, evidence and arguments, a process of constructive and civil 'knowledge exchange' between people occupying different positions, and procedures for collectively questioning, debating and testing evidence and arguments so as to ensure that decision making is informed by the fullest possible attention to relevant factors and perspectives. 'Accountability for reasonableness', the influential approach to priority setting cited in Chapter One, sits within this broad tradition of work and, in particular, explicitly draws on the key ideas that normatively underpin deliberative democracy. That is, that deliberation should be centred on reasons that can be recognised as relevant (even when not shared or accepted) by people who are 'fair-mindedly' informing and participating in the deliberation and should involve procedures that allow this full set of relevant reasons to emerge, be reviewed and be given due weight or 'fair consideration'.[3] These approaches cannot get around the problem that there are deep-seated and principled disagreements about what should be done and that practical decision making involves various kinds of compromise that will seem wrong-headed and unacceptable to some participants. On the contrary, they start from the recognition of these challenges and seek to address them in the best available way.

So we can assume that the overall governance of health systems, in particular, formal healthcare services, will continue to be led by representatives (sometimes elected) at various levels and it is, of course, likely that such representatives will be (to varying degrees) sensitive to indicators from populations – whether these are crude service quality data relating to 'satisfaction' or 'patient experience' and so on or political articulations and manifestations of discontent. But, in addition, I am arguing that even where formal deliberative democratic methods are not embraced or deemed practicable, that representatives, along with institutional leaders, will be energetically seeking and calling upon much richer forms of participation and data about people's perspectives, priorities and reasoning, and in particular will be requiring service providers to provide evidence of analogous ongoing dialogue with service users. This latter – the encouragement of meaningful dialogue with multiple constituencies of patients and families (for example, within different condition groups, service divisions, institutions, departments, clinics and so on) about what matters and about the merits and demerits of practices, as part of the process of organising and enacting care – is, I am arguing, essential for good healthcare. It is not merely an aspect of evaluating the quality of care; it is, for all the reasons rehearsed above, a necessary condition of being able to provide good care.

'Dialogue' is being used here as shorthand to point to a range of possibilities that can be supported by, but that also themselves contribute to, forms of patient, professional and public education. These include mutual listening and respect but also elements of collective deliberation and negotiation, which will sometimes mean dissent, contestation and some overt conflict. Activist movements, for example, can be influential while being in tension with, and not incorporated into, mainstream policy processes. The philosophical transition in health policy does necessitate and foster a more deliberative and democratic spirit, but this is much more than a tidy devolution of knowledge and responsibility.

Indeed it means taking seriously and trying to make practical, at least in part, some of the fuller aspirations of democracy: people coming together and making things together, debate and argument, and criticality and subversion. This might sound like an idealistic aspiration, and at times be very untidy and uncomfortable,[4] but within specific contexts (for example, interested system actors – both providers and users – working within specific domains to reshape relationships and practices) it can also be quite realistic.

Those with special responsibilities

The diffusion of expertise and responsibility, and the partial erosion of boundaries between policy makers and professionals, on the one hand, and publics and patients, on the other, creates new demands and dilemmas for the former, who have 'special accountabilities' for health and healthcare. First, before I discuss these demands and dilemmas, I want to suggest that we need to check ourselves when using terms like 'policy makers' and 'professionals' – do we know or agree whom we are referring to by these terms? If many more people are not just 'health actors' but also 'policy actors' (as is consistent with 'policy enactment theory', referred to in Chapter Five), then the category of policy maker becomes less clear cut and potentially misleading or exclusionary. Similarly we need to be careful about assuming that it is adequate to refer to 'professionals' or 'practitioners' – even on relatively elastic or liberal interpretations of these terms. There is an expansion in the numbers of, and recognition of, people – paid and unpaid, part time and full time – who have some kind of caring or practice role within the health and social care 'workforce', and there is a continual development of new kinds of roles.

Nonetheless there are some groups of actors – policy makers and professionals for short – who are 'answerable' for their health-related work in 'special' ways; that is, in ways that are relatively unqualified and are formalised because they are attached to specific roles and institutional frameworks. Most notably they belong to occupationally regulated groups and/or are nominated, elected or appointed into roles of leadership or service in government (at any level) or regulated public, private or voluntary organisations. Whereas each one of us is ethically answerable – albeit often in unclear and disputed ways – for our health-related acts and omissions, such people have formally recognised institutional, ethical and legal duties to provide good healthcare and, in many cases, to contribute to healthy environments. In more participative health systems, necessarily incorporating widespread dialogue, including exercises in collective deliberation and action, these dedicated roles become harder and the associated responsibilities more onerous.

To start with health professionals, where the changed demands are already being acknowledged – they can obviously no longer rely on the idea that they are the undisputed locus of expertise and authority. Rather than relying on deference, they increasingly have to earn respect and trust based on their ways of relating, including the manner in which they use their own insights and experience and are responsive to the insights and experience of others. Yet, at the same time, they retain substantially greater accountability for these processes and for decisions and outcomes than do patients and families. This is practically, intellectually and ethically highly challenging. It rests on (for some) new kinds of facilitation and communication capabilities, allied with value literacy including sensitivity to the way clinical, life-trajectory and value judgements are co-constitutive of one another. It involves being genuinely respectful and responsive to the things that matter to patients, and creating a supportive environment to enable these things to emerge, while being unafraid to question and debate (gently or robustly, depending upon people's characteristics and what is at stake) the issue of what is for the best, or to make recommendations or insist on 'red lines' in relation to what they are personally prepared to do or endorse.

Although it is less often highlighted, much the same is true for policy makers if their work is to be ethically defensible and not counter-productive. Certainly they have accountabilities of their own that they need to take seriously. But these accountabilities can be discharged only if their work is firmly based on ongoing dialogue and debate with professional and patient groups. All attempts to impose top-down edicts, unless these are genuinely emergent from habits of collective deliberation, will not simply be unethical and undemocratic but will inevitably be intrinsically ineffective – they will be directed and calibrated blindly. This is to note something much more important than the fact that professionals and others do not like to be told what to do and that such measures will likely be resisted and subverted in practice (although this is also true). It is, rather, a consequence of the main point of this chapter. A paradigm of 'delivery' is often unfit for purpose and, at best, is insufficient. Nowadays, to do health policy means to fully engage with people's perspectives and values – including the perspectives and values of 'providers'; otherwise there is no understanding of what is being done, or of the nature of healthcare. (To believe the opposite is the equivalent of believing that no knowledge of either music or fingering is needed for flute playing.)

Of course policy makers have imperatives and constraints of their own and, as with professionals, they will sometimes have high levels of access to sources of relevant knowledge and experience that provide good grounds for ruling out certain courses of action or for advocating others. In this context it is understandable that policy makers may choose to describe some of their decisions as 'evidence based'. But this is defensible only to the extent that those who make this claim manifest a clear understanding that (a) 'evidence' is only one factor in a cocktail of considerations that include arguments about purposes, principles and priorities; and (b) what counts as evidence is typically framed by these other factors and may be reasonably contested by other policy interlocutors. With these qualifications noted, policy makers may sometimes have grounds to make unpopular decisions and draw 'red lines' of their own. But, I am arguing, for their authority to be either effective or legitimate they need to demonstrate the same kind of respect for others that we have now come to expect practitioners to show to patients.

In short, this new climate for both professionals and policy makers – in which 'delivery' makes sense only in the context of engagement, dialogue and co-production – necessitates not only literacy about other people's perspectives and values but the capability to manage conflicts between perspectives and to understand, live with and self-consciously address normative dilemmas.

Expansive learning for new healthcare architectures

The trends I have been reviewing require us to develop partnerships between community members and those with special accountabilities that both embody mutual support and provide a platform for deliberation and policy making (along with the accompanying tensions and disagreements). As stressed in the last chapter, building these forms of partnership depends upon public and professional education, including upon taking advantage of the learning opportunities that arise as people from different vantage points come together to co-produce and enact new healthcare approaches. The idea that we require a 'learning healthcare system' is apposite here. However, this idea needs to be interpreted in an expansive way. Typically, the term 'learning healthcare system' is used to talk about the utilisation of digital technology, data monitoring and analytics to provide ongoing feedback into quality-improvement ambitions.[5] There is no need to side-line this highly promising line of work – as we have seen, it makes sense to place new digital possibilities at the centre of forward-looking thinking. However, I would suggest that this digital ambition will be a truly powerful one only if it is combined with the ambition of bringing together all community assets and partners for mutual learning. The learning needed would be expansive in multiple senses: entailing a very broad conception of relevant kinds of expertise (encompassing both relational and normative expertise); operating with a fluid notion of where expertise sits, including who are the teachers and the learners; oriented to persons in their full depth – their practices, dispositions and emotions and not just cognition in a narrow sense (for this dimension of expansiveness see Lucas et al, 2013); and, finally, requiring that expectations and practices of mutual learning are embedded and naturalised across the whole system. In various places I have summarised the educational and cultural change needed at an individual level in terms of changes to ways of seeing and ways of thinking, often involving significant gestalt switches. Such learning includes changes to what Charles Goodwin calls 'professional vision' (Goodwin, 1994), which is both supported by and consists in transformative learning. This includes the capacity to 're-see' something familiar in radically new ways – what is foregrounded might turn into background or vice versa (that is, with the 'figure' and 'ground' altering) – for example, to see patients as co-producers and co-citizens and not as a burden of care; or to clearly see the potential chasm between personalised medicine and personalised care.

In this context of partnership working the traditional logics of markets, bureaucracies and conventional professionalism are clearly insufficient and need to be both complemented and disrupted by other more democratically inspired forms of social coordination (the ground I have covered has resonances with numerous currents, including, for example, emancipatory social movements, community organising, civic and democratic inflections of professionalism and versions of social enterprise). I am suggesting that in forging new forms of social partnership the ideals and controversies surrounding rich forms of shared decision-making at an individual level provide – albeit by analogy – some guidance. The task is to jointly rethink and rework the nature of both healthcare relationships and healthcare decision making. In some respects the challenging situation that Freida faced in Chapter One – being positioned as a co-architect of the services she also relies upon – has to be generalised but somehow made manageable. Yet the challenge here is much broader than thinking about specific priority-setting dilemmas and entails both revisiting our conception of 'resources' and confronting – or at the very least making explicit – the philosophical balancing acts that run through health policy. Drawing on the arguments of this book I will try to sketch out this agenda a little further.

Policies, whether these are far reaching or quite local, cannot always be optimal for each party that is affected by them and sometimes people with quite legitimate expectations will fail to have these expectations met because of the balance of effects seen across other individuals and groups. This is familiar from the arena of resource allocation but is actually a much more widespread and deep-seated phenomenon. It is not just that health services must provide a particular 'package' of medicines, operations or other treatments and options and not a contrasting package, but that they will also embody a particular 'package' of normative assumptions and social and institutional dispositions and not, simultaneously, a contrasting package. Every actor, and especially policy makers and professionals, is constantly involved in the process of shaping this 'value package' – whether they recognise this or not – and they can do this more or less consciously, thoughtfully and defensibly. In other words, all health-policy debates must not only accommodate the question of what 'goods' should be provided by a health system but also the question of what count as 'goods' in this context – how goods are conceived, and how they can and should be realised and balanced together, including whose perspectives and voices should matter.

The implications of this for workforce and resource planning and for the preparation of professionals and other health and social care workers are substantial. For a start, these things – especially if we are to embrace something like 'asset-based' working – cannot be approached on the principle of 'more of the same'. Yes, it is true that attention needs to be paid to whether there are going to be 'enough' doctors and nurses and so on, but this mind-set (as another symptom of the delivery paradigm) can easily lead us in completely the wrong direction. At least as much thought needs to be given to (i) reimagining what is sometimes called the 'skill mix' in healthcare, not least the possibilities of self-care, peer support and community action, along with the development of new or extended professional roles that can enable and enact aspects of responsiveness to persons and care integration; (ii) expanding and strengthening the spaces – whether physical or digital, old or new – that enable people to come together and work together in both planning and realising care; (iii) refreshing and strengthening concepts of 'professionalism' (including for roles not traditionally thought of as professional roles) so that practitioners – at least a critical mass of them – combine sufficient clinical expertise with the forms of 'relational' expertise needed to successfully work in facilitative, collaborative and creative ways.[6] Such conceptions of good practice and extended professionalism must also reflect the fact that the normative discourses that shape agendas are framed by some interests and agents more than others, and actively consider how to support the kinds of 'protection' for vulnerable or disadvantaged persons that are familiar from one-to-one relationships.

More generally, we need to substantially reframe debates about 'resources'. This includes (but, as will shortly be discussed, extends beyond) the need to take 'disinvestment' seriously; in other words, facing up to the challenge that in some cases expenditure might need to be 'switched' from one area to another. However, this challenge, in itself, raises a vitally important and troublesome set of questions – constitutional and political questions about health-system boundaries and decision-making legitimacy; and practical and ethical questions about whatever is 'not done' – the impacts and ethics of disinvestment. However good the arguments might be for not doing certain things, such arguments are still very difficult to advance in democratic climates where multiple constituencies and vested interests have a voice and – for good reasons – expect to be heard. But in many cases there will be people who 'lose out' (even if only sometimes marginally) and who will, understandably, present themselves as being 'sacrificed' for the greater good. There are no easy answers to that objection. This is one of the reasons why I highlighted and praised Daniel Callahan's critique of technological medicine as the 'beloved beast' in Chapter Two. Callahan's analysis is particularly praiseworthy because he squares up to the conclusion that moves towards a more defensible healthcare system mean not only doing things differently but also stopping things that are valuable to some. And one thing does not cancel out the other. However, having stressed that, it should also be said that effectively mobilising large numbers of people as healthcare actors, as discussed in this chapter (and as was anticipated by many of the original critics of medicalisation), could substantially help to reduce wasted expenditure and expand the 'real resources' available for health and social care.

In other words, and most importantly, there is the need to reconceptualise the idea of 'resources' and detach it from the 'means–ends' technicist kinds of rationality, alluded to above, that often dominate healthcare thinking. Although I am uneasy about routinely describing human beings in economic terms, one of the benefits of the language of 'asset-based' thinking is that it underlines the fact that 'persons' are, for the most part, both the ends and the means of healthcare. If we hold this notion vividly in our minds we are bound to move away from the dominant emphasis of thinking of resources in terms of money or budgets. This includes, above all else, dropping the background assumption that resources are neutral assets that do not themselves constitute healthcare and can be transferred interchangeably between interventions. The further along the road we move in shifting the balance between biomedical models and person-centred models of healthcare, the more crucial it becomes to drop this assumption.

Socially oriented currents and conceptions of healthcare make huge resource demands and at the same time highlight and offer similarly huge resource possibilities. Person-centred healthcare calls, for example, for indefinitely large quantities of attention and compassion and – assuming that the relational and public dimensions of persons are properly recognised – collaboration and solidarity. At the same time communities can also, if mobilised effectively, provide untold quantities of these foundational goods. But the crucial thing to note here is that these goods are foundational in a strong sense – that is, they are themselves *constitutive* of healthcare.

To the extent that we come to understand resources in person-centred ways we cannot treat them as neutral assets – the fundamental nature and potential of healthcare is shaped by the way we think about and treat 'human resources' – including professionals, patients and broader communities. It now widely accepted that we cannot treat patients as objects or instruments but that good practice (judged in terms of both ethics and effectiveness) is completely dependent upon their being treated with respect. In the case of professional–patient relationships, for example, it is now commonplace to see that policy and practice can be creative or destructive with respect to the personal resources of patients – it can make people relatively 'fit for' or 'unfit for' shared decision-making, self-management or participation more generally. A regime that is in many respects conscientiously trying to use resources efficiently can quite easily – if it interprets this goal too narrowly – be both wasting and degrading resources in calamitous ways.

It is, more slowly, coming to be recognised that the same applies to professionals and other carers who are too easily treated as objects or instruments in processes of policy 'implementation' – something that is inherently degrading and counter-productive. Respect builds healthcare from the inside out; and disrespect – conscious or otherwise – destroys it in the same way. This insight – that the use and treatment of resources (including financial resources) is not neutral but shapes future possibilities – often in self-generating or self-destructive ways – applies at every level. After all, policy actors and carers are also patients; and patients are also carers and policy actors. Health policy needs to start from the recognition that health systems help to shape the persons who, in turn, shape health systems and enact healthcare.

Overall, I have been suggesting that health policy needs to embrace an expansive conception of learning and an enlarged conception of reasoning – one that incorporates technicist knowledge and rationality but that firmly sets these in the context of dialogue, deliberation and philosophical argument. Part of that reframing is to provide a counter-weight to the tendency to treat policy decisions in isolation from one another. This includes giving ongoing attention to debates about the architecture of health systems and health ecologies, including the building blocks – both ideas and their socio-material factors – from which they are made. Attention to these architectures is, as was concluded in Chapter Six, the core wisdom lying behind the justified rise of the notion of 'integration' up the health policy agenda. This is a generalised version of the conclusion I drew about Freida's priority-setting dilemmas in Chapter One. Individual evaluations cannot be made effectively without some sensitivity to our competing visions of the kinds of society we are trying to shape, and the balancing acts that have to be accomplished in the process.

In this book I have tried to outline some of the key balancing acts needed – the pervasive questions about the right balances between 'cure' and 'care', or biomedical and social emphases – and to highlight the myriad day-to-day judgements that are involved in cashing these balances out in practice. And bound up with these are debates about the best way to both arbitrate between and combine together different underlying models or logics of healthcare. This demands critical thinking about the ontology and epistemology of healthcare – what structures and relationships are constitutive of good healthcare, and what and whose expertise help to determine that. In other words, my argument is that health policy has now turned into a philosophical (as well as a scientific and social scientific) field. The contention here is broader and much more fundamental than simply saying that it has become a field in which philosophers are taking an interest. The claim is that the questions that are now central to the development of health policy and the evaluation of healthcare are inherently philosophical ones. As a consequence, policy makers, practitioners and all interested parties must roll up their sleeves and be prepared to get their hands dirty with the uncertainties and contestation that are now integral to health policy and practice.

This means, as I have tried to set out, wrestling with the implications of (competing) discourses of person-centred care and not assuming that these are either easily compatible with, or simply incompatible with, professionalised biomedicine. It means being ready to welcome ever more effective and 'precise' medical solutions, providing that we balance that welcome with an awareness of health as a social good: how do medical interventions cohere with, reinforce or undermine the many other ways in which health and well-being can be promoted? Are medical and other interventions properly anchored in an understanding of what matters to people understood collectively or individually? We also need to find a balance between causal and narrative forms of understanding – are the structures and relationships we are building doing justice to both? Finally, while recognising that persons are interconnected and that individuals and populations cannot be neatly contrasted – are we striking the right balance between underpinning a health ecology and system that protects and supports the broader common good, including public health and interventions that predominantly reflect and serve the interests of particular individuals? These – I am suggesting – are the key issues that must be consciously and continuously balanced and debated within official policy making, and by all interested policy actors, and should inform and animate specific decisions about design and provision.

Conclusion

Health-policy discourses have evolved so as to redraw the relationships between 'medicine' and 'persons'. Social lenses – along with very many associated normative and relational questions and concerns – are now at the heart of healthcare thinking. As a consequence, intelligent policy making and analysis has to be ready to focus on persons (in all their diversity and complexity) as both the ends and means of healthcare, and on the social conditions that underpin their health and well-being, including by differentially enabling (or disabling) them as health actors. This inevitably takes health policy into challenging and marshy territory. The more we understand health and healthcare, the more we come to see that there is very little reassuringly solid ground to stand on. But this discovery need not be alarming – rather, we should remember that if we are genuinely pursuing effective and equitable healthcare, then there is an obligation to be sceptical about authoritative-looking knowledge claims. In the process, what may be lost by way of certainty and confidence will be replaced by gains in responsiveness and – in the fullest sense – by gains in rigour as well.

Notes

1   See, for example, NHS England's Healthy New Towns programme – https://www.england.nhs.uk/ourwork/innovation/healthy-new-towns/.

2   Taking Charge of Health and Social Care, Greater Manchester Combined Authority – see links from www.gmhsc.org.uk/news/publichealthplanforgreatermanchester/.

3   This notion that all relevant reasons should be appraised fairly is, arguably, implicit in the accountability for reasonableness approach, but it has been recently argued by Rand that this is insufficient and that it should be made an explicit condition of it (see Rand, 2016).

4   For example, see Jane McGrath's (2016) illuminating account of both the frustrations and successes of trying to make co-production work in practice.

5   Institute of Medicine, The Learning Health System Series (cited 5 January 2016). Available from: www.nap.edu/catalog/13301/the-learning-health-system-series.

6   There is clear evidence that some of the implications of the ongoing healthcare transition for professional education – for example, capabilities for partnership working and for a broader repertoire of professional styles of working and relating – are recognised within official policy circles (see, for example Health Education England, 2014). But the full breadth of the implications of the more expansive learning models needed is thus far only patchily accommodated across the breadth of education and healthcare institutions.

References

Atkinson, P. (1995) *Medical talk and medical work*, London: Sage.

Ball, S., Maguire, M. and Braun, A. (2011) *How schools do policy*, London: Routledge.

Bambra, C. (2016) *Health divides: Where you live can kill you*, Bristol: Policy Press.

Barber, N. (1991) Is 'safe, effective and economic' enough? *Pharmaceutical Journal*, 246, 671–2.

Batalden, M., Batalden, P., Margolis, P., Seid, M., Armstrong, G., Opipari-Arrigan, L. and Hartung, H. (2015) Coproduction of healthcare service, *BMJ Quality and Safety*, doi: 10.1136/bmjqs-2015-004315.

Bohman, J. and Rehg, W. (1997) *Deliberative democracy: Essays on reason and politics*, Cambridge, MA: MIT press.

Bridges, D., Davidson, R., Soule Odegard, P., Maki, I. and Tomkowiak, J. (2011) Interprofessional collaboration: three best practice models of interprofessional education, *Medical Education Online*, 16, 6035, doi: 10.3402/meo.v16i0.6035.

Caldwell, J.C. (1993) Health transition: the cultural, social and behavioural determinants of health in the Third World, *Social Science and Medicine*, 36, 125–35.

Callahan, D. (2009) *Taming the beloved beast: How medical technology costs are destroying our health care system*, Princeton, NJ: Princeton University Press.

Carter, S., Rogers, W., Heath, I., Degeling, C., Doust, J. and Barratt, A. (2015) The challenge of overdiagnosis begins with its definition, *BMJ: British Medical Journal (Online)*, 350:h869, doi: 10.1136/bmj.h869.

Charles, C., Gafni, A. and Whelan, T. (1997) Shared decision-making in the medical encounter: what does it mean? (Or it takes at least two to tango), *Social Science and Medicine*, 44, 681–92.

Coulter, A. (2016, 1 July) At last some better news on shared decision making, *The BMJ Opinion* [Online]. Available: http://blogs.bmj.com/bmj/2016/07/01/angela-coulter-at-last-some-better-news-on-shared-decision-making/ [Accessed 7 April 2017].

Coulter, A. and Collins, A. (2011) *Making shared decision-making a reality*, London: The King's Fund.

Cragg, L., Davies, M. and Macdowall, W. (eds) (2013) *Health promotion theory (Understanding public health)*, Maidenhead: Open University Press.

Cribb, A. and Entwistle, V.A. (2011) Shared decision making: trade-offs between narrower and broader conceptions, *Health Expectations*, 14, 210–19.

Cribb, A. and Gewirtz, S. (2015) *Professionalism*, Cambridge: Polity Press.

Cribb, A. and Owens, J. (2010) Whatever suits you: unpicking personalization for the NHS, *Journal of Evaluation in Clinical Practice*, 16, 310–314.

Cribb, W. (2015) *Telegram from Mandalay*, Lytham St Annes: Inkstand Press.

Daniels, N. (2000) Accountability for reasonableness in private and public health insurance, *British Medical Journal*, 321, 1300–1.

Denford, S., Frost, J., Dieppe, P. and Britten, N. (2013) Doctors' understanding of individualisation of drug treatments: a qualitative interview study, *BMJ Open*, 3, e002706, doi: 10.1136/bmjopen-2013-002706.

Denford, S., Frost, J., Dieppe, P., Cooper, C. and Britten, N. (2014) Individualisation of drug treatments for patients with long-term conditions: a review of concepts, *BMJ Open*, 4, e004172, doi: 10.1136/bmjopen-2013-004172.

Donetto, S. and Cribb, A. (2011) Researching involvement in health care practices: interrupting or reproducing medicalization? *Journal of Evaluation in Clinical Practice*, 17, 907–12.

Du Gay, P. (2000) *In defence of bureaucracy*, London: Sage.

Edwards, A. and Elwyn, G. (2009) *Shared decision-making in health care: Achieving evidence-based patient choice*, Oxford: Oxford University Press.

Engel, G. (1977) The need for a new medical model: a challenge for biomedicine, *Science*, 196, 129–136.

Entwistle, V. and Cribb, A. (2013) *Enabling people to live well: Fresh thinking about collaborative approaches to care for people with long-term conditions*, London: The Health Foundation.

Entwistle, V.A., Cribb, A. and Owens, J. (2016) Why health and social care support for people with long-term conditions should be oriented towards enabling them to live well, *Health Care Analysis*, doi: 10.1007/s10728-016-0335-1.

Entwistle, V., Firnigl, D., Ryan, M., Francis, J. and Kinghorn, P. (2012) Which experiences of health care delivery matter to service users and why? A critical interpretive synthesis and conceptual map, *Journal of Health Services Research and Policy*, 17, 70–8.

Fotaki, M. (2014) *What market-based patient choice can't do for the NHS: The theory and evidence of how choice works in healthcare*, London: Centre for Health and the Public Interest.

Frankfurt, H. (1982) Freedom of the will and the concept of a person. *In:* Watson, G. (ed.), *Free will*, Oxford: Oxford University Press.

Frankl, V. (2004) *Man's search for meaning*, London: Ebury Publishing.

Fraser, N. (1996) Social justice in the age of identity politics: Redistribution, recognition and participation, *The Tanner Lectures on Human Values*, Stanford University, 30 April–2 June [Online]. Available: http://tannerlectures.utah.edu/_documents/a-to-z/f/ Fraser98.pdf [Accessed 7 April 2017].

Fraser, N. (2013) *Fortunes of feminism: From state-managed capitalism to neoliberal crisis*, London: Verso.

Freidson, E. (2001) *Professionalism, the third logic: On the practice of knowledge*, Chicago: University of Chicago Press.

Germov, J. (2005) Managerialism in the Australian public health sector: towards the hyper-rationalisation of professional bureaucracies, *Sociology of Health and Illness*, 27, 738–58.

Giddens, A. (1991) *Modernity and self-identity: Self and society in the late modern age*, Cambridge: Polity Press.

Gilbert, T.P. (2005) Trust and managerialism: exploring discourses of care, *Journal of Advanced Nursing*, 52, 454–63.

Glasziou, P., Moynihan, R., Richards, T. and Godlee, F. (2013) Too much medicine; too little care, *British Medical Journal*, 347:f4247, doi: https://doi.org/10.1136/bmj.f4247.

Goffman, E. (1961) On the characteristics of total institutions, *Symposium on preventive and social psychiatry*, Walter Reed Army Medical Centre Washington, DC, 43–84.

Goodwin, C. (1994) Professional vision, *American Anthropologist*, 96, 606–33.

Graham, H. (2009) *Understanding health inequalities*, Maidenhead: Open University Press.

Greenway, J.C. and Entwistle, V.A. (2013) Ethical tensions associated with the promotion of public health policy in health visiting: a qualitative investigation of health visitors' views, *Primary Health Care Research and Development*, 14, 200–11.

Habermas, J. (1987) *The theory of communicative action Vol 2. Lifeworld and system: A critique of functionalist reason*, Boston, MA: Beacon Press.

Harris, S. (2005) Professionals, partnerships and learning in changing times, *International Studies in Sociology of Education*, 15, 71–86.

Health Education England (2014) *Framework 15: A Health Education England strategic framework 2014–2029* [Online], London: Health Education England. Available: https://hee.nhs.uk/sites/default/ files/documents/HEE%20Strategic%20Framework%20-%20 Framework%2015.pdf [Accessed 7 April 2017].

Heggie, V. (2013, 5 May) *What's killing us: Statistics, tuberculosis and the McKeown thesis* [Online]. Available: https://www.theguardian.com/science/the-h-word/2013/mar/05/mortality-statistics-mckeown-history-tuberculosis [Accessed 7 April 2017].

Hellawell, B. (2016) Partnership working and the SEND code of practice 2015: Policy enactment and policy ethics. Doctoral thesis, King's College London.

HMSO (2013) *Report of the Mid Staffordshire NHS Foundation Trust Public Inquiry*, London: The Stationery Office.

Horne, R., Weinman, J., Barber, N., Elliot, R., Morgan, M., Cribb, A. and Kellar, I. (2005) *Concordance, adherence and compliance in medicine taking*. Report for the National Co-ordinating Centre for NHS Service Delivery and Organisation, London: NCCSDO.

Illich, I. (1976) *Limits to medicine*, London: Marion Boyars Publishing.

Kaur, J. and Mohanti, B.K. (2011) Transition from curative to palliative care in cancer, *Indian Journal of Palliative Care*, 17, 1–5.

Kodner, D.L. and Spreeuwenberg, C. (2002) Integrated care: meaning, logic, applications, and implications–a discussion paper, *International Journal of Integrated Care*, 2, doi: http://doi.org/10.5334/ijic.67.

Komesaroff, P.A. and Rothfield, J.D. (1997) *Reinterpreting menopause: Cultural and philosophical issues*, London: Routledge.

Le Grand, J. (2007) *The other invisible hand: Delivering public services through choice and competition*, Princeton, NJ, Princeton University Press.

Lucas, B., Claxton, G. and Spencer, E. (2013) *Expansive education: Teaching learners for the real world*, Maidenhead: Open University Press.

Lupton, D. (1997) Foucault and the medicalisation critique. *In:* Petersen, A. and Bunton, R. (eds), *Foucault, health and medicine*, London: Routledge.

MacIntyre, A. (2007) *After virtue: A study in moral theory*, Notre Dame, IN: University of Notre Dame Press.

Mackenzie, C. and Stoljar, N. (eds) (2000) *Relational autonomy: Feminist perspectives on automony, agency, and the social self*, Oxford: Oxford University Press.

McGrath, J. (2016, 31 October) Co-production: an inconvenient truth? *The King's Fund* [Online]. Available: https://www.kingsfund.org.uk/blog/2016/10/co-production-inconvenient-truth? [Accessed 7 April 2017].

McKee, M. and Stuckler, D. (2012) The crisis of capitalism and the marketisation of health care: the implications for public health professionals, *Journal of Public Health Research*, 1, 236–9.

Marmot, M. (2015) *The health gap: The challenge of an unequal world*, London: Bloomsbury Publishing.

Milbourne, L., Macrae, S. and Maguire, M. (2003) Collaborative solutions or new policy problems: exploring multi-agency partnerships in education and health work, *Journal of Education Policy*, 18, 19–35.

MIND (2016) *Our communities, our mental health: Commissioning for better mental public health* [Online]. Available: www.mind.org.uk/ media/2976113/mind_public-mental-health-guide_web-version. pdf [Accessed 5 January 2017].

Mladenov, T., Owens, J. and Cribb, A. (2015) Personalisation in disability services and healthcare: a critical comparative analysis, *Critical Social Policy*, 35, 307–26.

Mol, A. (2008) *The logic of care: Health and the problem of patient choice*, London: Routledge.

Mooney, G. (2012) *The health of nations: Towards a new political economy*, London: Zed Books.

Morgan, H.M., Entwistle, V.A., Cribb, A., Christmas, S., Owens, J., Skea, Z.C. and Watt, I.S. (2017) We need to talk about purpose: a critical interpretive synthesis of health and social care professionals' approaches to self-management support for people with long-term conditions, *Health Expectations*, 20, 243–59.

Morrison, M. and Glenny, G. (2012) Collaborative inter-professional policy and practice: in search of evidence, *Journal of Education Policy*, 27, 367–86.

Mulley, A., Trimble, C. and Elwyn, G. (2012a) Patients' preferences matter. *Stop the silent misdiagnosis*, London: The King's Fund.

Mulley, A., Trimble, C. and Elwyn, G. (2012b) Stop the silent misdiagnosis. Patients' preferences matter, *British Medical Journal*, 345:e6572. http://www.bmj.com/content/345/bmj.e6572.

Navarro, V. (2009) What we mean by social determinants of health, *Global Health Promotion*, 16, 5–16.

NIH National Cancer Institute (2016) *NIH National Cancer Institute's guidance on BRCA1 and BRCA2 testing* [Online]. Available: www. cancer.gov/about-cancer/causes-prevention/genetics/brca-fact-sheet [Accessed 7 April 2017].

Nuffield Council on Bioethics (2010) *Medical profiling and online medicine: The ethics of 'personalised healthcare' in a consumer age*, London: NCOB.

Osborne, S.P., Radnor, Z. and Nasi, G. (2013) A new theory for public service management? Toward a (public) service-dominant approach, *The American Review of Public Administration*, 43, 135–58.

Osborne, S.P., Radnor, Z. and Strokosch, K. (2016) Co-production and the co-creation of value in public services: a suitable case for treatment? *Public Management Review*, 18, 639–53.

Owens, J. and Cribb, A. (2012) Conflict in medical co-production: can a stratified conception of health help? *Health Care Analysis*, 20, 268–80.

Parrott, L. (2008) The ethics of partnership, *Ethics and Social Welfare*, 2, 24–37.

Parsons, T. (1951) *The social system*, Glencoe, IL: The Free Press.

Pereira Gray, D., White, E. and Russell, G. (2016) Medicalisation in the UK: changing dynamics, but still ongoing, *Journal of the Royal Society of Medicine*, 109, 7–11.

Prainsack, B. (2017) *Personalized medicine: Empowered patients in the 21st century?* New York, NY: New York University Press.

Rand, L. (2016) Legitimate priority-setting: refining accountability for reasonableness and its application with NICE. Unpublished PhD thesis, Oxford University.

Ranmuthugala, G., Plumb, J.J., Cunningham, F.C., Georgiou, A., Westbrook, J.I. and Braithwaite, J. (2011) How and why are communities of practice established in the healthcare sector? A systematic review of the literature, *BMC Health Services Research*, 11, 273, doi: 10.1186/1472-6963-11-273.

Rippon, S. and Hopkins, T. (2015) *Head, hands and heart: Asset-based approaches in health care*, London: The Health Foundation.

Rose, N. (1989) *Governing the soul: The shaping of the private self*, London: Routledge.

Royal College of Psychiatrists (2010) *No health without public mental health: The case for action (Position statement PS4/2010)* [Online], London: Royal College of Psychiatrists. Available: www.rcpsych. ac.uk/PDF/Final%20PS4%20briefing_for%20website%20A4.pdf [Accessed 7 April 2017].

Sandel, M.J. (2012) *What money can't buy: The moral limits of markets*, London: Penguin Books.

Schwartz, B. (2004) *The paradox of choice: Why more is less*, New York, NY: Harper Collins.

Sellman, D. (2011) *What makes a good nurse: Why the virtues are important for nurses*, London: Jessica Kingsley Publishers.

Smith, R. (2015, 2 February) Is the NHS being the top issue in the election a sign of a degenerate society? *The BMJ Opinion* [Online]. Available: http://blogs.bmj.com/bmj/2015/02/02/richard-smith-is-the-nhs-being-the-top-issue-in-the-election-a-sign-of-a-degenerate-society/ [Accessed 7 April 2017].

Taylor, C. (1992) *The ethics of authenticity*, Cambridge, MA: Harvard University Press.

Thomas, R. (2002) *Society and health*, New York, NY: Kluwer Academic Publishers.

Thompson, D.F. (2008) Deliberative democratic theory and empirical political science, *Annual Review of Political Science*, 11, 497–520.

Tones, K. and Tilford, S. (2001) *Health promotion: Effectiveness, efficiency and equity*, Cheltenham: Nelson Thornes.

Toon, P. (2014) *A flourishing practice?* London: Royal College of General Practitioners.

Topol, E. (2015) *The patient will see you now: The future of medicine is in your hands*, New York: Basic Books.

Vackerberg, N., Levander, M.S. and Thor, J. (2016) What is best for Esther? Building improvement coaching capacity with and for users in health and social care – a case study, *Quality Management in Health Care*, 25, 53–60.

Wade, D. (2009) Holistic healthcare, what is it, and how can we achieve it? Presentation to the Nuffield Orthopaedic Centre AGM.

Wennberg, J.E. (2010) *Tracking medicine: A researcher's quest to understand health care*, Oxford: Oxford University Press.

White, K. (2016) *An introduction to the sociology of health and illness*, London: Sage.

Wolff, J. and De-Shalit, A. (2007) *Disadvantage*, Oxford: Oxford University Press.

Index

A

accountability for reasonableness 24, 173–4
activation, and shared decision making (SDM) 57–60
agency *see* patient agency
asset-based working 162–3, 180–1
autonomy 50–1, 59–60, 65–6, 67, 72, 171
　see also patient agency

B

BBC news report 117, 118
bed-blocking 133–4, 134–5
biomarkers 109
biomedical model 29–38
　digital health 163–9
　and patient agency 72–6
　and technology 41–2
　see also medicalisation
biopsychosocial model of health 81
BMA 117
bureaucracy 93–4

C

Callahan, D. 39–41, 180
care
　concept of 7–9
　and patient agency 70–2
　personalised care 120–8
Carter, S. 43
choice *see* patient agency
collective responsibility 169–75
common good 40, 64–5, 69, 88, 122
consistency of treatment 91–5
consumerism 66–9
coordination *see* integration
cure, idea of 7–9
cyberspace 163–9

D

Daniels, N. 24
de-medicalisation 29–34, 38
decision-making
　collective responsibility 172–4
　decision support tools 74–5
　shared decision-making (SDM) 57–66, 72, 73–5, 110–12
deliberative democracy 173–4
delivery paradigm 154
democratisation 160–9
　deliberative democracy 173–5
Denford, S. 111–12
digital health 163–9
　concerns about 165–7
discrimination 83–4, 94–5
disinvestment 180
doctors *see* health professionals
Du Gay, P. 93–4

E

Edwards, A. 58
effectiveness, clinical 21–3, 25, 46–7, 77
efficiencies 95–101
Elwyn, G. 58
epidemiological transition 5–6
Esther Project Network 136–7
evidence 21–5
evidence-based medicine (EBM) 59–60
evidence-based patient choice (EBPC) 57–60
expansive learning 177–82
expenditure *see* healthcare expenditure
expertise/experts 175–7
external and internal goods 100–1

F

feminist critiques 33
Fotaki, M. 69

Foucault, M. 34, 67
Francis Inquiry report 98–9
Freidson, E. 35

G

genetic testing 108–9
Glasziou, P. 45
Goffman, E. 82
Goodwin, C. 178
Greater Manchester, Health and Social
  Care Partnership 172

H

Habermas, J. 99–100, 149
Harris, S. 146
health, concept of 20–1
Health and Social Care Partnership
  (Greater Manchester) 172
health inequalities 28, 79–80, 89, 96,
  166–7
health policy
  health promotion 85–91
  policy futures 14–24
  re-balancing 47–53, 178–80
  trends 10–13
  unbalanced 38–47
health professionals
  and cyberspace 168
  and holism 91–5
  and integration 137–49
  and medicalisation 34–8, 41–2
  professionalism 35–7, 60, 68, 91
  reconceputalising of relationships 159
  and shared decision making (SDM)
    57–66, 72, 73–5, 110–12
  and special responsibilities 175–6
  see also patient agency; personalisation
health promotion 48, 85–91
health transition 5–6
healthcare expenditure
  disinvestment 180
  efficiencies 95–101
  wasted 38–41
hierarchy of needs 48, 49
holism 79–102
  and depersonalisation 81–4, 99–101
  and efficiency 95–101
  and exclusion 83–4
  external and internal goods 100–1
  and Habermas 99–100
  and health promotion 85–91
  interpretations of 81–5
  and organising clinical care 91–5
  personal vs social 81–4
Hopkins, T. 162–3

I

iatrogenesis 32, 36, 43–4
Illich, I. 32
information sharing 143–4
Institute of Medicine 24
institutionalisation 82–4
integration 129–51
  challenges of 142–51
  common professional framework
    144–9
  divisions and boundaries 130–4
  Esther Project Network 136–7
  health and social care 137–42
  hypothetical case studies 134–7
  information sharing 143–4
  need and potential for 134–7
  processes of 148
  realigning relationships 137–42
inter-professional working 144–9

K

Kodner, D.L. 140–1

L

Lupton, D. 34

M

MacIntyre, A. 100
marketisation 41–2, 66–8, 97, 155
McKeown, T. 33
media, and personal health budgets
  117–18
medical profession see health professionals
medicalisation 29–34
  critiques of 32–4, 42–3
  extension of 41–2, 110
  feminist critiques 33
  moving beyond 34–8
  over-diagnosis 42–3, 44–6
  and personalised medicine 110
  and power 34
medicine, model of 34–7
methodological individualism 88, 169
Mid Staffordshire Trust 98–9
Mol, A. 70–2
mutually agreed tailoring (MAT) 112

N

need 23
  hierarchy of needs 48, 49
new professionalism 60
non-compliance 48–9

O

Osborne, S.P. 125, 126
outputs 22–3
over-diagnosis 42–3, 44–6
over-treatment 40–1, 43–4

P

palliative care 9
partnerships 143–9, 177–82
path dependency 60–1
patient agency 55–77
    and autonomy 65–6
    and biomedicine 72–6
    broader controversies of 66–9
    and care 70–2
    challenges of 60–6
    choice of provider 68–9
    and collective responsibility 169–75
    and consumerism 66–9
    and decision support tools 74–5
    and democratisation 160–9
    and digital health 163–9
    evaluation of 63–4
    evidence-based patient choice 57–60
    and mental capacity 62–3
    and person-centredness 47–52
    and personalised medicine 110–12
    scope of 62–3
    shared decision making (SDM)
    57–66, 72, 73–5, 110–12
    tensions within 64
Pereira Gray, D. 41–2
person-centredness 47–52
    see also patient agency; personalisation
personal health budgets 113–20
personalisation 103–28
    concept of 103–8
    and digital health 163–9
    dimensions of 105–8
    divergences of interpretation 105–8,
    111–12
    and health equity 107–8
    personal health budgets 113–20
    personalised care 105–6, 120–8
    personalised medicine 105–6,
    108–13, 127–8
    see also patient agency
personalised care 105–6, 120–8
personalised medicine 105–6, 108–13,
    127–8
philosophical transition in healthcare 5–7
policy makers, and special responsibilities
    176–7
    see also health policy
power, and medicalisation 34
practice variations 43, 58–9

P (continued, right column)

Prainsack, B. 167
precision medicine 109
priority setting 14–19
    comparing value 19–24
product logics 125–6
professionalism 35–7, 60, 68, 91
    see also health professionals
public goods 88
Pulse 117, 120

R

Radnor, Z. 125, 126
relational autonomy 65–6
resources 180–1
respect for patient autonomy (RPA)
    59–60
Rippon, S. 162–3
Rose, N. 67

S

Schwartz, B. 66
scientific-technological basis 35–6
screening programmes 44–5
second-order desires 90–1
self-management 76, 146–7
    digital health 163–9
    see also personalisation
service logics 125–6
shared decision making (SDM) 57–60
    and biomedicine 73–5
    and care 72
    and personalised medicine 110–12
    problems with 60–6
Smith, R. 27
social determinants of health 3
social goods, healthcare as 156–60
Spreeuwenberg, C. 140–1

T

targeting of health promotion 87, 89–90
Taylor, C. 103
technological mindset 41–2
technology, and the future 163–9
    see also medicalisation
Topol, E. 163, 164
total institutions 82–4
trade-offs 13–19

W

Wade, D. 81
Wennberg, J.E. 43, 59